marie claire

hair & makeup

ACKNOWLEDGEMENTS

I would like to thank Catie Ziller for her ongoing support and for believing in me from start to finish with this project, and Anne Wilson, Jackie Frank and Matt Handbury for the opportunity to develop the concept. Special thanks to Debbie Pike for her endless enthusiasm, outstanding creativity and, most importantly, her great friendship. Thanks to David Parfitt for his innovative photography, brilliant eye and hours of hard work, and to Troy Word for his energy, creativity and ability to capture the spirit of this book on film. Special thanks also to Linda Hay for all her amazing make-up and to Tim Crespin for his great hairdos. To models Glenna, Melissa, Kim, Susan, Audrey and Carolyn for all your help and enthusiasm; to my editor, Lesley Levene, for making sense of this all and always being so calm; to my sister, Susie, for her endless support, drive and for keeping me sane—I couldn't have done this book without you; and to Stewart for the laughs that kept me going, to Brenda for her inspiration and to Brian for always being so level-headed, and to all my friends, especially Nicola, Nicky, Brendan and Sam and Michael, for being so understanding and supportive while I've been working on this book.

10 9 8 7 6 5 4 3 2 1

Published in 2003 by Hearst Books,
A Division of Sterling Publishing Co., Inc.
387 Park Avenue South, New York, NY 10016

Originally published in 1998 by Murdoch Books
© Text Jane Campsie 1998.
© Design and photography Murdoch Books® 1998.
Text edited by Didi Gluck and Genevieve Monsma

Marie Claire is a trademark of, and is used under license from, Marie Claire Album. Hearst Books is a trademark owned by Hearst Communications, Inc.

www.marieclaire.com

Distributed in Canada by Sterling Publishing
C/o Canadian Manda Group, One Atlantic Avenue, Suite 105
Toronto, Ontario, Canada M6K 3E7

ISBN 1-58816-278-8

Library of Congress Cataloging-in-Publication Data

Campsie, Jane.
   Marie Claire hair & makeup / Jane Campsie.
      p. cm.
   Includes index.
   ISBN 1-58816-278-8
   1. Beauty, Personal. 2. Hair--Care and hygiene.
3. Cosmetics--Popular works. I. Title: Marie Claire hair and makeup. II. Title: Hair & makeup. III. Title.
   RA778.C2153 2003
   646.7'2--dc21
                                                    2003006315

marie claire

hair &
makeup

JANE CAMPSIE

Still-life photography: David Parfitt   Beauty photography: Troy Word

HEARST BOOKS
Sterling Publishing Co., Inc.
NEW YORK

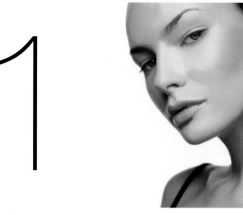
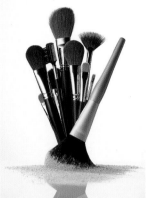
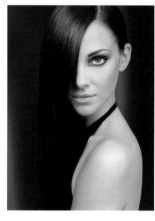
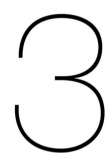
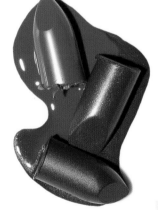
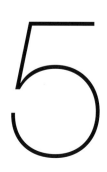
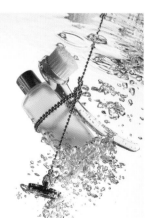

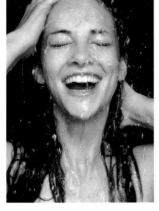

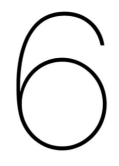

6

HAIR MAINTENANCE
the best regimen for you and your hair 108

7

PREP WORK
make sense of hair products 128

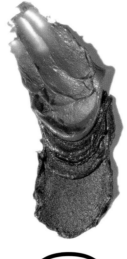

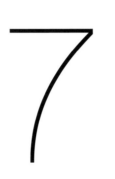

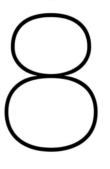

8

CREATIVE SOLUTIONS
master the art of hairstyling 144

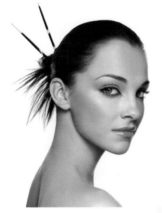

9

HAIR COLOR
the lowdown on hair color 158

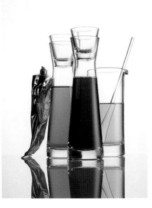

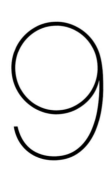

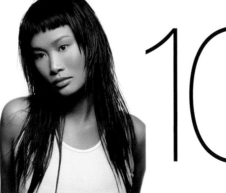

10

EXPRESS BEAUTY
high-speed hair and makeup 172

GLOSSARY
186

INDEX
187

PHILOSOPHY

marie claire hair & makeup offers a realistic approach to modern beauty to boost your self-esteem and confidence. It is not about following the latest make-up trends, wearing the color of the moment or sporting the most fashionable hairstyle. It is about adapting different looks to suit you, in order to accentuate your best features and bring out your natural beauty. So if you have never really experimented with different hairstyles and makeup or are stuck in a beauty rut and simply want a change, use this book to your advantage. There are no strict rules and regulations as to what you can and can't do when it comes to hair and makeup. The secret is to find what suits you and your lifestyle. In keeping with the pressures of modern living, it is essential to find ways to maintain hair upkeep and perfect your makeup quickly without cutting back on the results—all the time aiming to make looking good a simple task. I hope that you will find this book easy to follow and will reap the benefits, improving the way you look and feel and, most importantly, enjoying yourself in the process.

—Lesley Jane Seymour
Editor-in-Chief, *marie claire*

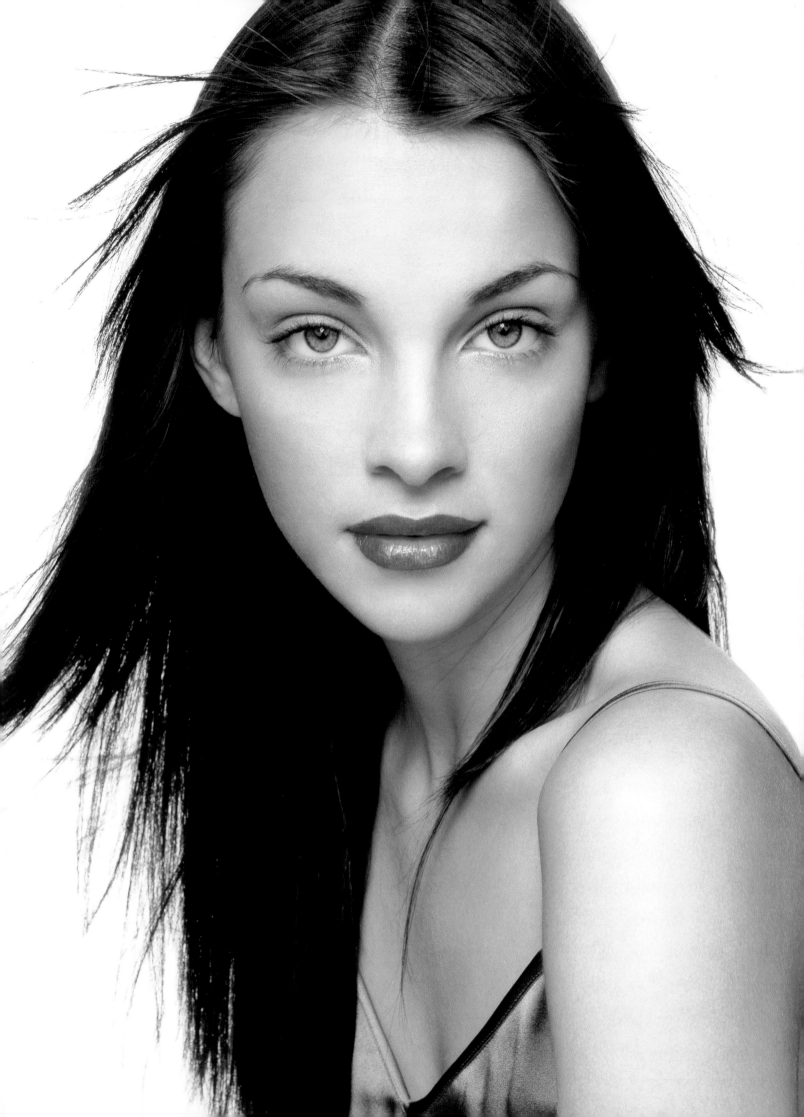

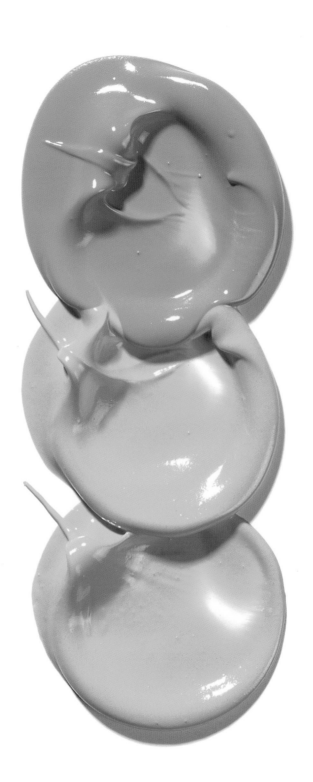

bare essentials

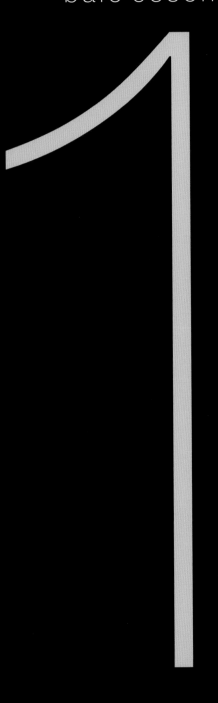

Makeup should be used to help you look good and feel better. Find your own basic makeup essentials to create a radiant-looking complexion and then experiment with different colors, textures and cosmetic items to accentuate your features and enhance your face. Improving your appearance will boost your confidence and self-esteem.

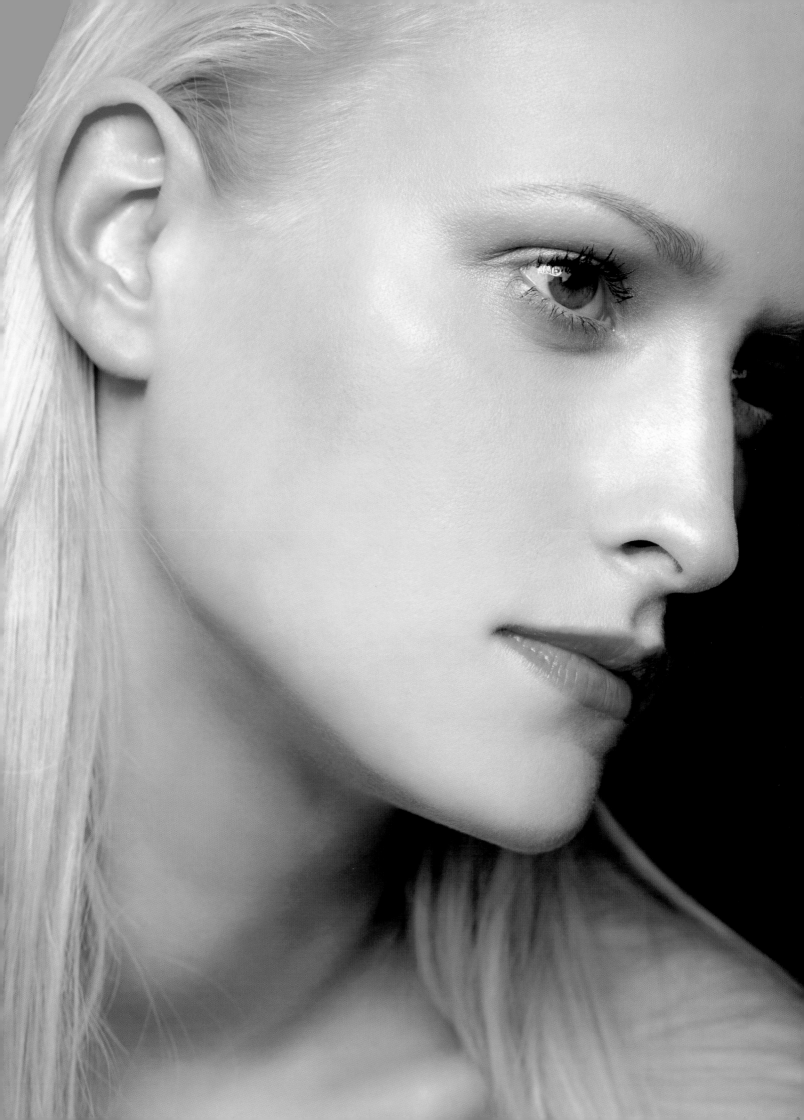

MAKEUP
ESSENTIALS

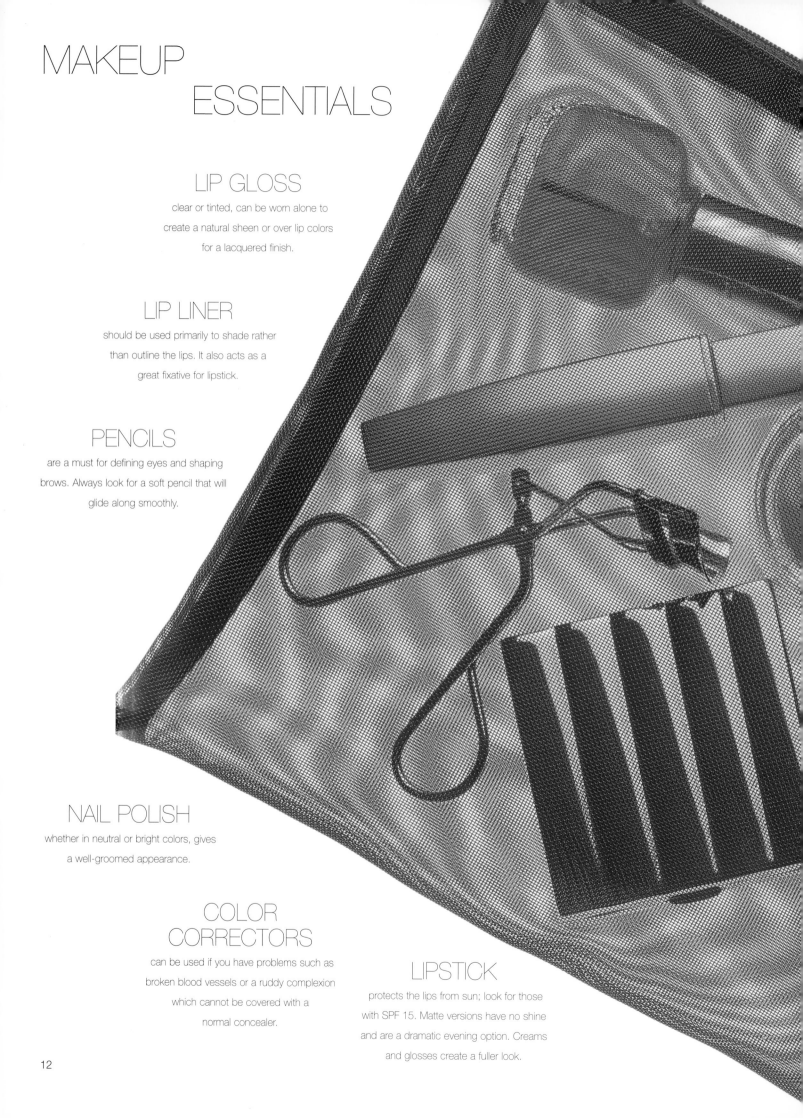

LIP GLOSS

clear or tinted, can be worn alone to
create a natural sheen or over lip colors
for a lacquered finish.

LIP LINER

should be used primarily to shade rather
than outline the lips. It also acts as a
great fixative for lipstick.

PENCILS

are a must for defining eyes and shaping
brows. Always look for a soft pencil that will
glide along smoothly.

NAIL POLISH

whether in neutral or bright colors, gives
a well-groomed appearance.

COLOR
CORRECTORS

can be used if you have problems such as
broken blood vessels or a ruddy complexion
which cannot be covered with a
normal concealer.

LIPSTICK

protects the lips from sun; look for those
with SPF 15. Matte versions have no shine
and are a dramatic evening option. Creams
and glosses create a fuller look.

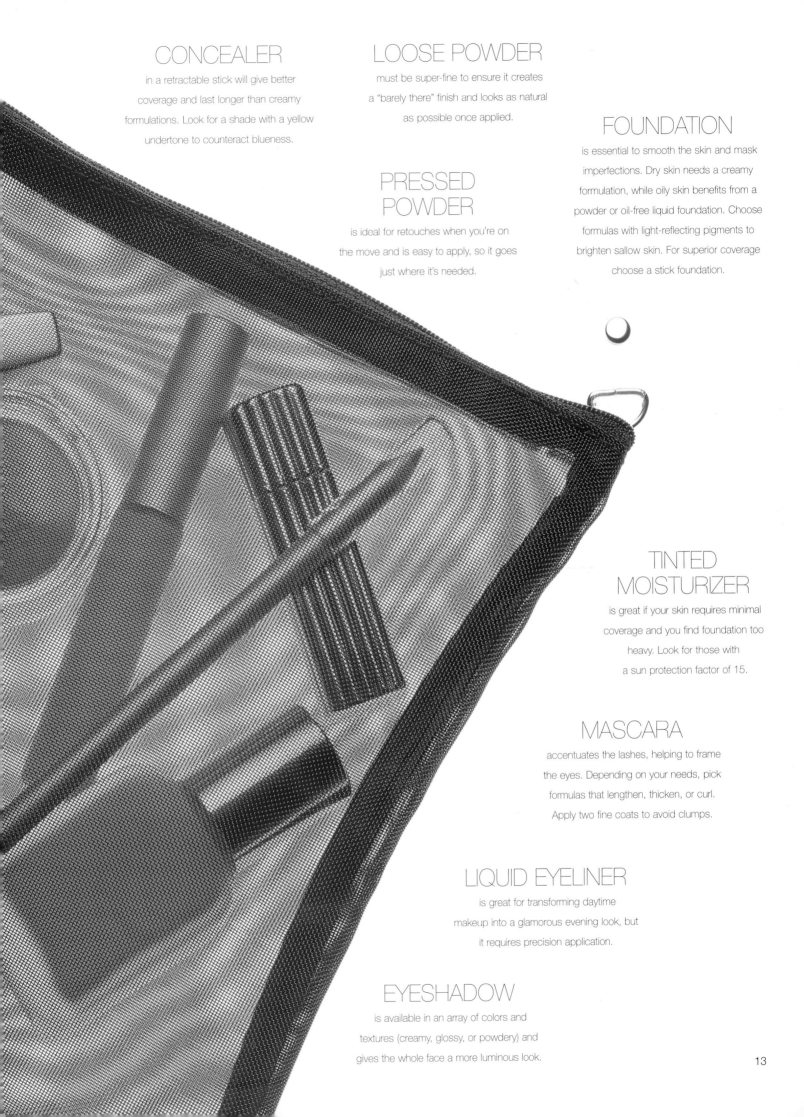

CONCEALER

in a retractable stick will give better coverage and last longer than creamy formulations. Look for a shade with a yellow undertone to counteract blueness.

LOOSE POWDER

must be super-fine to ensure it creates a "barely there" finish and looks as natural as possible once applied.

PRESSED POWDER

is ideal for retouches when you're on the move and is easy to apply, so it goes just where it's needed.

FOUNDATION

is essential to smooth the skin and mask imperfections. Dry skin needs a creamy formulation, while oily skin benefits from a powder or oil-free liquid foundation. Choose formulas with light-reflecting pigments to brighten sallow skin. For superior coverage choose a stick foundation.

TINTED MOISTURIZER

is great if your skin requires minimal coverage and you find foundation too heavy. Look for those with a sun protection factor of 15.

MASCARA

accentuates the lashes, helping to frame the eyes. Depending on your needs, pick formulas that lengthen, thicken, or curl. Apply two fine coats to avoid clumps.

LIQUID EYELINER

is great for transforming daytime makeup into a glamorous evening look, but it requires precision application.

EYESHADOW

is available in an array of colors and textures (creamy, glossy, or powdery) and gives the whole face a more luminous look.

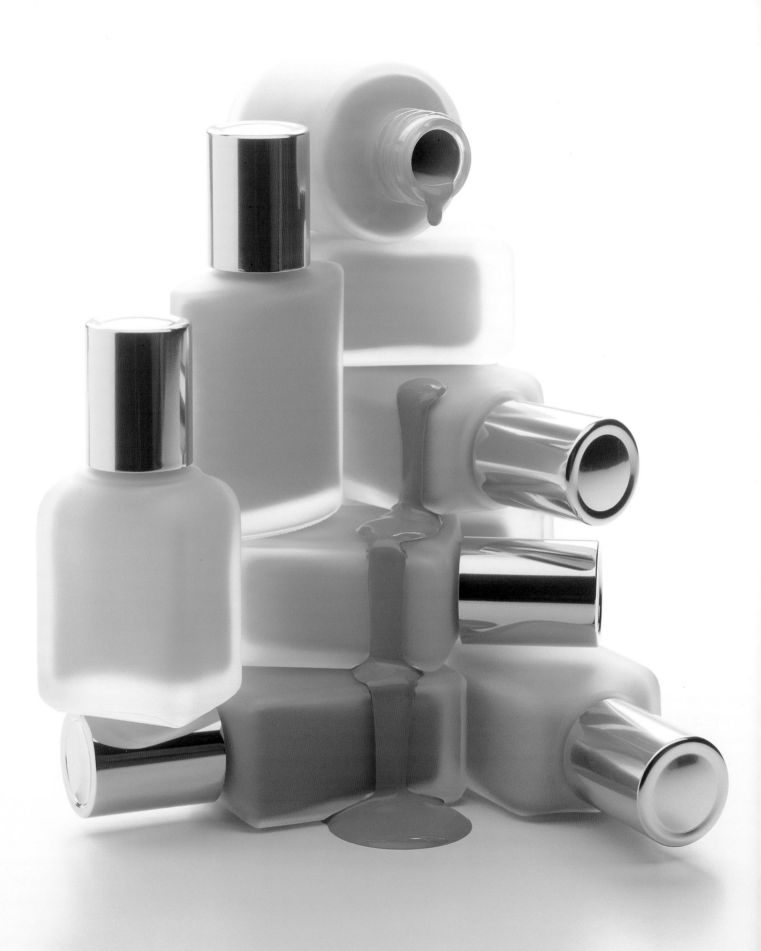

BASE
WORK

FOUNDATION Applied properly, foundation can make any complexion seem healthy and flawless. The aim is to leave the skin looking as natural and un-madeup as possible. Before you start, think hard about your complexion, as you may not need to apply base over the entire face. When choosing a foundation, take into consideration your skin type, the amount of coverage you require and the kind of finish you are after. And remember, you wear foundation every day, so making the right investment at the beginning will pay off.

FORMULATIONS Different foundations will provide different types of coverage. Stick formulas can be applied with the fingertips or a sponge, giving sheer to medium coverage. For the best results, smooth on in fine layers, gradually building up. It is much easier to add makeup than try to remove it after application. Compact foundations combine face powder and foundation in one. They are usually creamy formulations which dry to a matte finish and are available in oil-free versions. Some can be applied wet with a damp makeup sponge to achieve greater coverage, or with a dry sponge for a more natural-looking finish. Compact foundations are a great option if you're pushed for time as they're fast and easy to apply. Liquid foundations give good coverage and come in different finishes. Tinted moisturizers and sheer formulations give minimal coverage, making them ideal for younger skins. Mineral foundations, which usually come in a loose-powder form but can also be found in a compact, are a great option for those with sensitive skin, as they contain no chemicals (they're made from crushed minerals.)

SKIN TYPES If you have sensitive skin, look for formulations that do not contain potential irritants such as fragrance, chemical sunscreens and alpha hydroxy acids. Mature, dry skins will benefit from rich, creamy foundations which contain emollients to boost the skin's moisture content and antioxidants to protect it from environmental damage. Oily, problem skins will benefit from oil-free formulations, enriched with oil absorbers to keep unsightly shine at bay. Normal skins can wear any sort of foundation. In hot, humid weather, every skin type will benefit from an oil-free foundation.

SHOPPING FOR FOUNDATION To find the perfect foundation for your particular coloring, apply three suitable shades in strips across the cheek and jawbone. You are looking for the one that literally disappears into the skin. Your foundation should blend with the skin tone of the neck and not the face, as this is where it has to work down to. If you can't find the correct color, custom-blended foundations are available. When you try a new shade, check it in natural light. You should always aim to apply your makeup in daylight. When trying a new foundation, always wait fifteen minutes before reaching a decision, as the oil on your skin and the air can combine to darken the shade you have chosen.

FOUNDATION ESSENTIALS When looking for a new foundation, bear in mind that it should contain a sun protection factor of at least 15 for daily use. If not, you should wear a separate sunscreen on top. This should then be increased in summer, as the sun is responsible for 90 percent of premature aging. Antioxidants will also help protect the skin from visible signs of aging. Light-reflecting pigments will give a flattering finish, taking attention away from any dark circles and sallow-looking areas while adding instant luminosity.

EXPERT ADVICE To apply foundation, start from the center of the face, dotting on to the cheeks and forehead and blending outwards, first making sure your fingertips or makeup sponges are spotlessly clean. Gently blot the skin with a tissue to remove any excess product or surface oil. Never drag the skin if you are using your fingertips to apply cosmetics. If you're not very good at blending foundation, try applying it with a makeup sponge or brush. After smoothing on, moisten the fingertips and then work over the neckline to remove any signs of haphazard application. Blending with a damp sponge will yield a sheerer finish.

UNDER COVER

CONCEALER If you do not have a flawless complexion, concealer will be one of the most valuable cosmetics in your quest for beauty perfection. It can be used to disguise broken capillaries, dark circles, pimples and blemishes, and to even out skin tone. For the best all-around coverage, opt for a stick concealer (creamy and liquid concealers can be oily and have a tendency to slide on and off, whereas stick formulas will stay put). The only drawback with them is that they can be more difficult to blend. To overcome this, work the stick up and down the back of your hand. The product will warm up, making it more pliable and so easier to use. Apply it with the fingertips so that it literally melts into the skin. Those with dry skin will need a concealer with emollients to counteract dryness, while those with oily, problem skin will need a concealer that is oil-free and contains antibacterial ingredients to help treat blemishes and spots.

SHADE SELECTION To counteract blueness and dark circles under the eyes, go for a concealer with a yellow undertone that is one to two shades lighter than the color of the skin itself. If concealer is being used to mask pimples, to even out skin tone or to tone down broken capillaries, ensure that the shade you choose has a yellow undertone (pinkish shades will only accentuate redness) and is a good match for the natural color of your skin. Makeup artists advise testing concealer shades on the inside of the forearm.

APPLICATION Always apply your concealer on top of foundation before you add powder. If you try to do things the other way around, you might wipe the concealer off when applying your foundation. To disguise under-eye darkness, gently pat concealer under the eyes using the index finger. Exert only gentle pressure and blend outwards, taking care not to drag the skin. To conceal bags under the eyes, put concealer on the shadow beneath the bag, not on the bag itself; otherwise you'll end up highlighting rather than hiding the problem. To cover up broken capillaries or uneven skin tone, you can either massage concealer into the skin or paint it on with a brush and blend with the fingertips. To hide any blemishes or spots, paint on concealer with a brush. Remember to start at the center of the imperfection and feather outwards.

PROBLEM SOLVERS If your concealer dries and cakes in fine lines and wrinkles around the eyes, try using an eye cream under the concealer; make sure you use only a small amount of concealer and opt for one with a matte finish to create the illusion of smooth skin. On the rest of your face, to prevent the concealer from highlighting a problem you're trying to hide, apply a light moisturizer as an undercoat. Allow it to soak in and then dab away any excess with a tissue. This will make the skin soft and more even to work on. For extra staying power, once you have applied concealer, especially over pimples, set with a light dusting of translucent powder. If concealed areas dry out and start to flake throughout the day, gently pat on a small amount of moisturizer.

COVERING SCARS Scars or birthmarks can be disguised using heavy-duty concealers. Concealers designed for television will give great coverage and are available in water-resistant and waterproof formulations to ensure they stay put in a range of different circumstances.

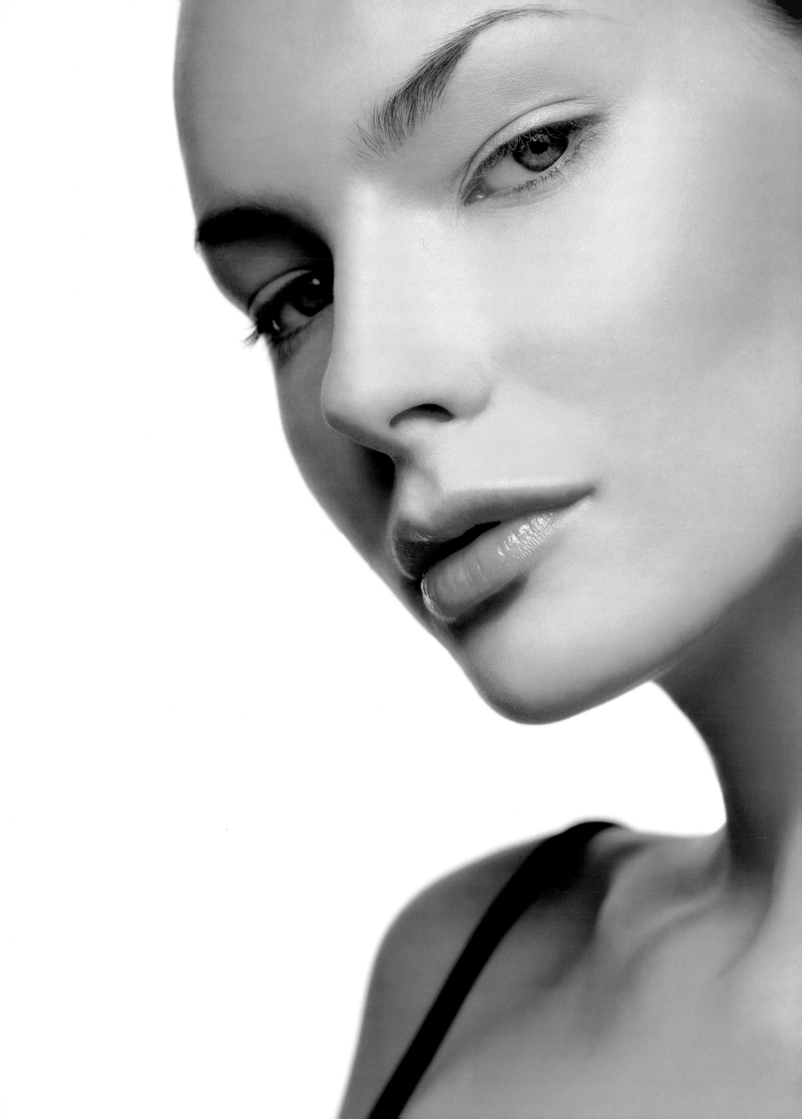

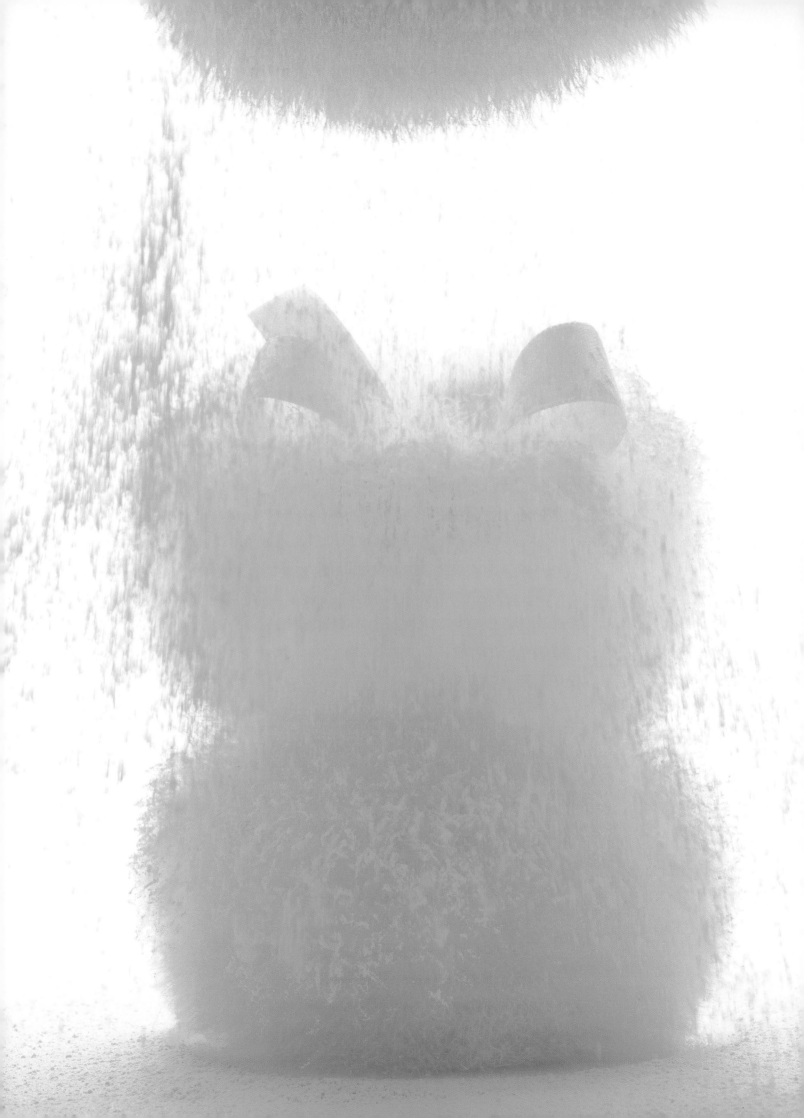

POWDER FINISH
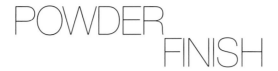

POWDER Face powder can be one skin type's ally and another's arch enemy. Oily skins will benefit from face powder that contains special oil-absorbing ingredients to give the skin a matte finish and will mop up unsightly oil secretions. After several hours' wear, if your skin starts to look shiny, blot it with a clean tissue to absorb excess surface oil and then touch up with face powder. If you have dry skin, go lightly with the powder; otherwise you will only accentuate the dryness. If you are using a foundation that aims to create a dewy-looking finish, avoid using any powder at all.

FORMULATIONS Decisions as to loose or pressed powder are a matter of personal preference. Loose powder is ideal to use when you're at home but is impractical to carry around, while pressed powder is great for retouches when you're on the move and is much easier to control. If you have a tendency to be heavy-handed when applying makeup generally, steer clear of loose powder.

COLOR CHOICE Opt for a totally translucent powder, or one that matches your foundation. Translucent powders are not, as most people imagine, invisible; they can zap the natural color of the skin and make complexions look chalky. To determine if a powder is good quality, test it on the back of your hand; it should feel silky and smooth and very light, and allow your natural coloring to come through.

APPLICATION Let your foundation settle for a couple of minutes before dusting on powder. There is no need to apply powder all over the face. Aim to keep your complexion looking as fresh and dewy as possible. Use powder mainly on areas of the face that are prone to shine, such as the chin, nose and forehead. For the best results when applying face powder, dust on with a brush in small swirling motions over the face and then sweep the brush downwards. This will remove any excess powder that has collected around the eyebrows or under superfluous facial hair and will ensure that these hairs lie flat on the face. If you want to use loose powder but are not confident about your ability to control the brush, try dusting the powder into the palms of your hands, then rubbing your hands together gently and pressing them over your face. Finally, run a large brush over your face to remove any excess powder.

EXPERT ADVICE Take a tip from the makeup artists: It is worth investing in a small natural sea sponge to use to set your makeup (they're available at beauty supply stores.) After applying your foundation and powder, press the damp sponge lightly into your complexion. This will make your base look fresh and dewy, instead of powdery and lifeless.

BRONZING POWDER To give the complexion a radiant glow, you can always use bronzing powder instead of face powder. Look for a bronzer which is one or two shades darker than your skin tone—but avoid shades which are too dark, as they will look very unnatural. For the best results, dust bronzing powder on the cheeks, tip of the chin, nose and forehead, and finish by sweeping over the entire face. Bronzers laced with flecks of shimmer can add luminosity to the complexion, but if you have older skin choose a matte version for a more flattering finish.

EYE COLOR

EYESHADOW This should always glide on smoothly, and can be used to subtly change or enhance the shape of the eyes, to add simple definition or to make a strong impact, depending on your choice of color. It is also useful to disguise the blueness many of us have on the skin of our eyelids.

CREAM VS POWDER Whether you wear cream or powder eyeshadow is a matter of personal preference. Cream-to-powder eyeshadows are easy to apply, as they can be swept over the eyelid in one stroke, but they have the disadvantage of gliding off again within hours of application or of creasing in the eyelid. To improve the staying power of cream eyeshadow, try setting it with a light dusting of translucent powder. While powder eyeshadows do tend to stay put, they require greater precision in application. Powder eyeshadows also flatter more mature skin.

COLOR CHOICE When you select colors, remember that dark ones deepen or hollow features, while light ones will make the eyes stand out. Choose bright colors carefully. They can look great but they draw attention instantly to the eyes and run the risk of looking unnatural, unless the face is balanced with other suitable makeup colors. Don't be put off by eyeshadow colors before you have tried them, as most will appear more intense in the palettes than they do on skin. Experiment with bright shades, but use them as a wash over the eyelids to add a subtle hint of color. You don't need to wear colors that match the color of your eyes, but it's a good idea to select shades which will accentuate your natural coloring. For those with blue eyes, try liner in brown or navy and avoid wearing blue eyeshadow. Green eyes stand out when shaded with khaki and brown shades with yellow undertones. Very dark brown eyes can wear almost any color but look especially striking with browns, charcoal and mahogany. Finally, grey/green eyes are enhanced by charcoal and black.

OPTICAL ILLUSION If you wear glasses, take into consideration the type of lenses you have when you are selecting makeup. If you are near-sighted, corrective lenses will magnify your eyes, so unless you have naturally small eyes wear muted or natural shades of eyeshadow. If you are far-sighted, your lenses will make your eyes appear smaller, so use eyeshadow to strengthen them. Dust eyeshadow along the socket line and outer corners of the eyes, but do not shade the eyelid heavily. Avoid wearing eyeliner on the upper lash line and steer clear of dark eyeshadow, as this will make the eyes appear smaller than they are. Also, frames will cast a shadow on the face, so disguise any darkness with a concealer one shade lighter than your foundation.

EXPERT ADVICE makeup artists recommend that when you are wearing eyeshadow, you should pile on extra loose powder under the eyes to catch any stray particles of eyeshadow. This can be removed by dusting off with a large makeup brush. After application, if you feel your choice of eyeshadow is too intense, tone the color down by dusting with face powder or gently wipe a foundation sponge over the eyelid to make the overall effect more subtle. To ensure that eyeshadow is long-lasting and crease-proof, makeup artists often apply a shadow base first. Another trick for helping powder color to stay on is to apply it with a damp brush. As the color dries, it will adhere to your skin—but use a light hand as this can also intensify the hue.

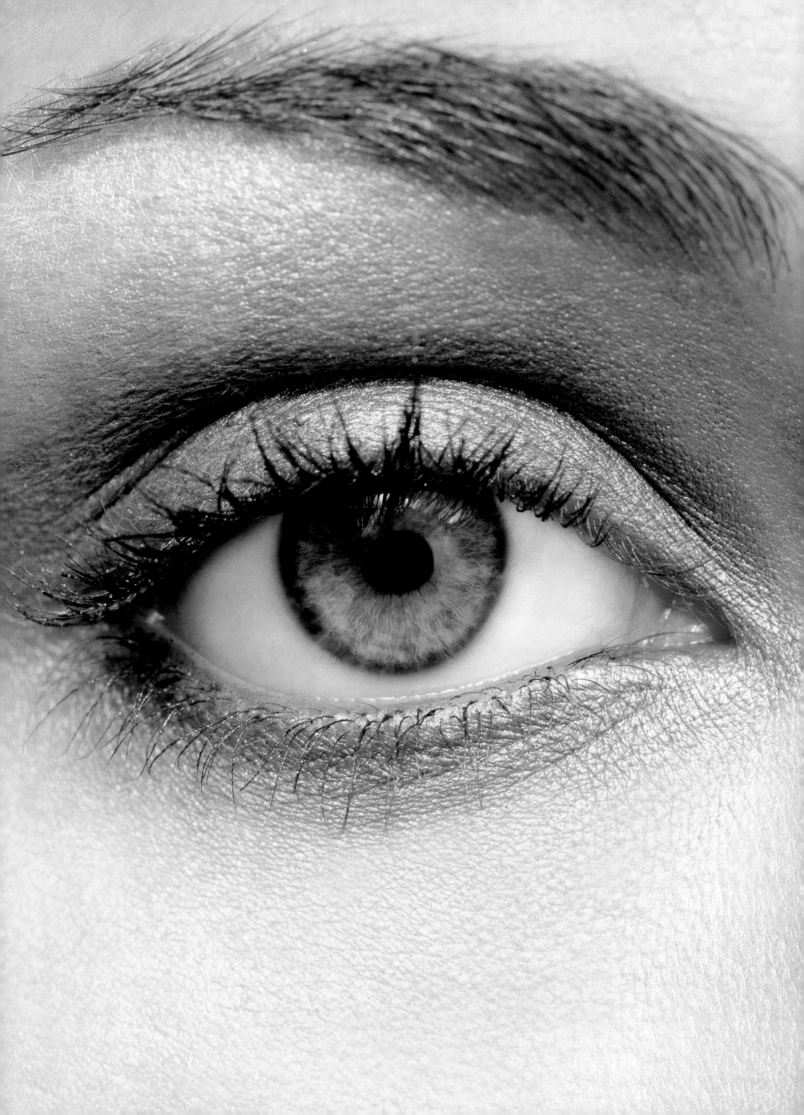

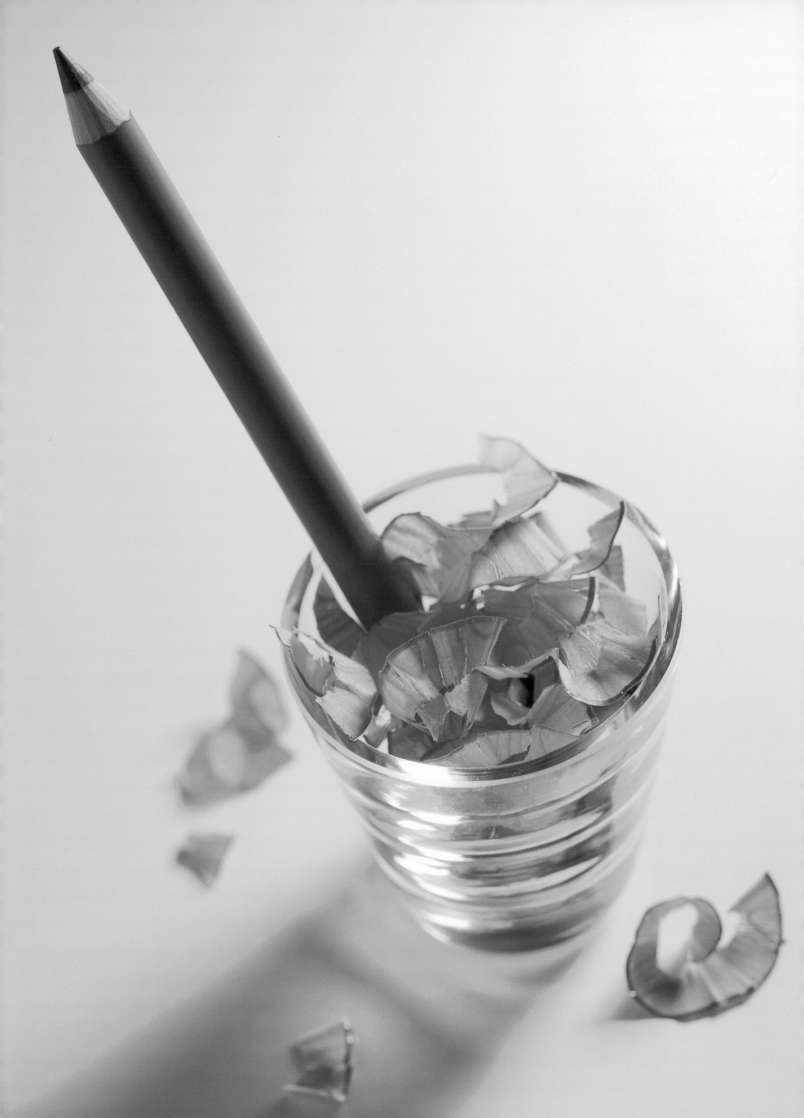

EYE DEFINITION

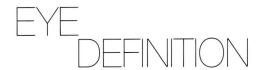

PENCILS Whether they are being used to shade or define the eyes, lips or brows, pencils should glide on smoothly, without dragging the skin. If they seem to be too soft and crumbly, place them in the freezer for a few minutes to harden before applying. If they are too hard and pull at the skin, soften the point first by gently running it over the back of the hand.

EYELINER Application requires a steady hand. If you find it difficult to apply liner with precision, try drawing it on using small feathered stokes and then blend with a fine-tipped brush or the point of a cotton swab. To make things easier, put a mirror on a flat surface and then work looking down into it. As an alternative to the visible pencil line on the eyes, try a connect-the-dots approach. Dot pencil between the lashes and then run over the dots with a fine-tipped brush. For an extra-defined look, dip an angled liner brush in water then use it to paint on eyeshadow in a thin line at the base of your upper lashes. It's worth investing in a white eyeliner: it could save the day on many occasions. If you're tired and your eyes don't look particularly sparkly, run a white pencil along the inner rim of the lower lash line. You will instantly look more awake and the whites of your eyes will appear brighter. It can also make small eyes appear larger. Never lend eye pencils to other people, as this is one of the quickest ways to spread germs. If you have an eye infection, replace eye pencils and mascaras to avoid reinfecting the eyes. Sharpen pencils regularly to ensure that the points are clean.

BROW PENCILS These can be used to fill sparse brows and enhance the overall shape. Take a sharpened pencil in the shade closest to the natural color of your eyebrows and fill any open spaces, using short irregular strokes to simulate real hair. When defining the brows, avoid drawing on one strong line as this will look fake. Work over the brows in small feathered strokes. If the definition is too strong, soften it by dusting with translucent powder or roll a cotton swab over the brows.

MASCARAS As mascaras are now loaded with proteins and waxes to condition the lashes and come in problem-solving formulations, look for one that suits your needs. Thin, sparse-looking lashes will benefit from lash-building formulations that contain special ingredients to add volume and thickness. If you wear contact lenses, do not use lash-building mascaras, as the fibers within them can get trapped between eye and lens, causing irritation. Short lashes should be coated with mascaras containing plastic polymers which cling just to the tips of the lashes to create the illusion of extra length. Sporty and outdoor types should opt for a waterproof or water-resistant mascara (the former will withstand a dip in the pool, while the latter holds up only to tears or perspiration).

WONDER WANDS However refined the formula, the shape of the mascara wand plays a significant role in lash definition. For example, crescent-shaped wands will help curve the lashes up; fat wands with lots of bristles will help thicken the lashes by coating each one individually; bristleless wands (they look like the tip of a metal screw) will allow you to paint lashes right to the roots; and double-tapered brushes (they have small bristles at either end that get longer towards the middle of the wand) will help define very thin and sparse lashes.

EXPERT ADVICE With modern mascaras there is no need to pump the wand in and out of its container before applying. This can actually cause overload and result in clogged lashes. You need only enough product on the wand to coat the lashes, so any excess should be wiped off with a tissue. Roll the wand through the lashes to help curl-definition. Always work on the upper lashes from underneath to avoid overloading and keep mascara on the lower lashes to a minimum, especially if you are looking tired or have a tendency to rub your eyes a lot.

LIP
FIX

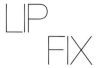

LIPSTICK This is one of the easiest and quickest ways to transform your appearance. You don't need to coordinate your lip color with your nail polish or wardrobe, but you may want to take into consideration what you are wearing. It is essential to ensure that your lip color blends with the rest of your makeup look and also complements your skin tone. Those with olive complexions should opt for colors with warm undertones to brighten the skin, such as light brown, raisin or brown reds, like blackberry and wine. Those with fair complexions need lip colors with warm peach or pink undertones, while those with pale complexions can wear almost any color, using dramatic shades to make a strong beauty statement. Dark complexions look best with deep reds with dark blue or purple undertones or deep browns with purple, blue or wine undertones.

FINDING THE FORMULATION To test-run a new shade, don't try it on the back of your hand. Instead, dab it on to your fingertip, where the color of the skin is closest to that of your lips. This can also be held near your mouth, to see if the color suits you. Once you have found the correct shade, you need to consider the effect you are after. Glossy finishes give sheer coverage but need to be reapplied frequently. Matte finishes give great coverage but have a tendency to be drying on the lips and can look very flat; to overcome this, look for demi-matte finishes, which dry to a more flattering finish. Creamy finishes create opaque coverage with a hint of shine and come enriched with conditioners, making them a suitable choice if your lips are prone to dryness. Sheer lipsticks give the lips a subtle wash of color, similar to lip gloss, but are longer-lasting. They are ideal as lightweight options to wear during the summer. Lip gloss has a tendency to slide off within hours of application. To help it stay put, prime the lips with a lip pencil in the shade closest to the natural color of the lips. Then apply gloss to the center of the top and bottom lip and purse the lips together. This creates the illusion of all-over shine without the problem of disappearing gloss.

EXPERT ADVICE If you want to wear a dark lipstick but doubt your application skills, use your fingertip and dab it on so the pigment stains the skin, then coat with lip gloss. To avoid leaving lipstick marks on glasses and cups, discreetly lick the rim before drinking. If lipstick always ends up on your teeth, place your middle finger in your mouth, pout and withdraw the finger. If you are pushed for time, avoid wearing dark or bright lipsticks as they need precision application and use gloss or a neutral-toned lipstick instead. If your lipstick has a tendency to bleed or feather into fine lines around the mouth, use a lip liner to shade the entire lip area before applying lipstick; also, wearing a lipstick that dries to a matte finish should help. Avoid wearing lipsticks with a frosted finish as you get older, since these will only highlight any lines around the mouth.

LIP PENCILS Do not use just to outline the lips—this looks very dated and you could be left with a unsightly line when your lipstick wears off—but to define and shade the entire lip area. This acts as a fixative for lipstick and ensures that your lip color will fade evenly. For a natural look, apply in a series of small feathered strokes around the outer edges of the lips, then blend with the fingertips and shade over the lips with the liner. If your lips are dry, making the liner hard to manoeuvre, coat them with lip balm first and blot with a tissue before applying. You do not need to buy different-colored lip liners to match different lipstick shades. Rather, choose one similar to your natural lip color and use this to shade and define the lips.

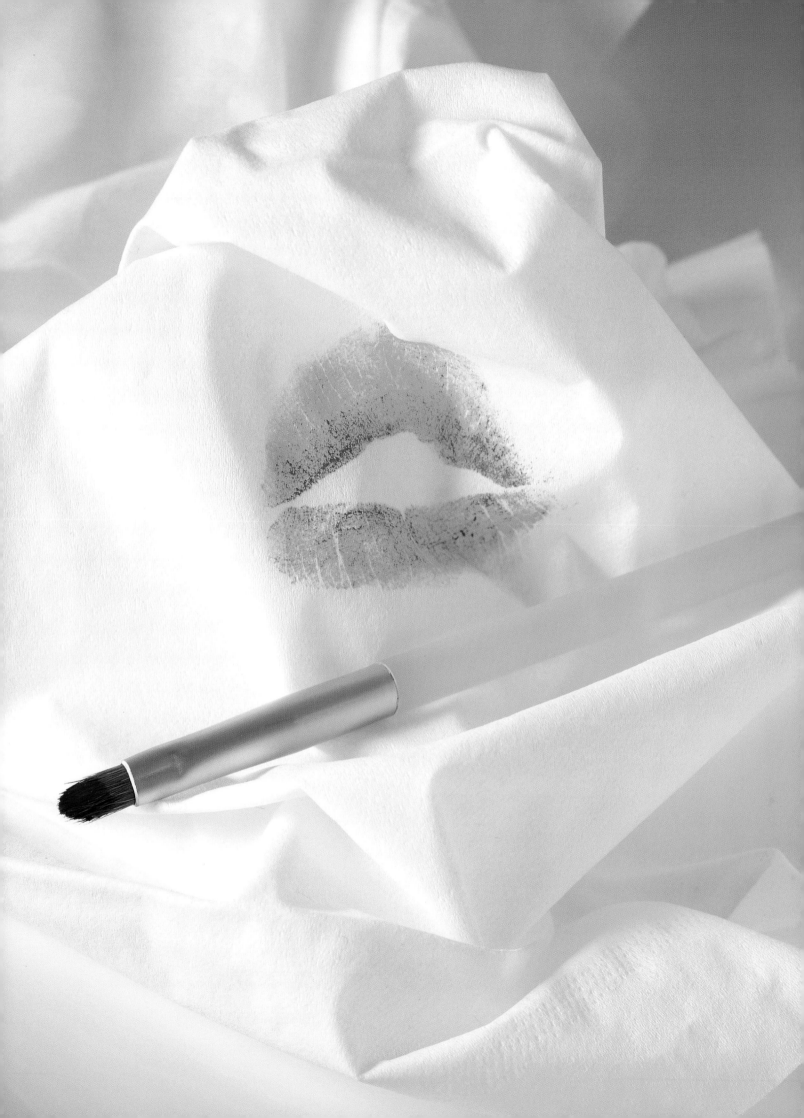

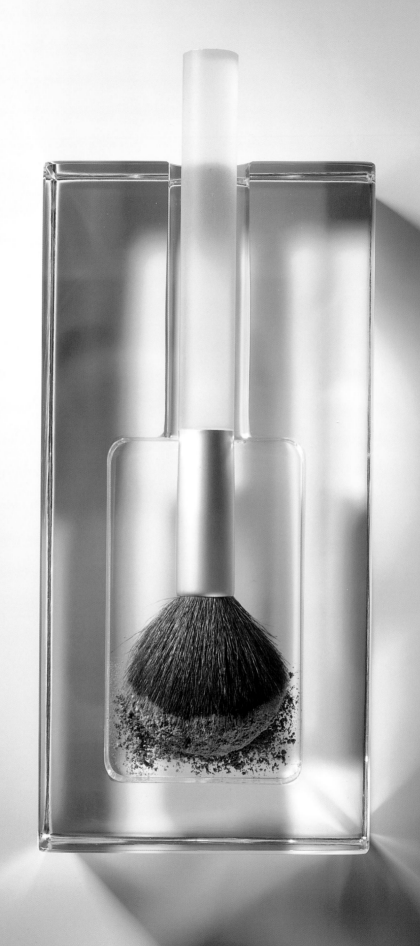

CHEEK COLOR

BLUSH If you haven't got razor-sharp cheekbones, don't worry: with the correct blush you can achieve anything. Whether you wear a powder or a cream blush, the secret is to create an effect which looks completely natural—unless, of course, you are going for the latest fashion look. With any cosmetic item, the choice between cream and powder formulations is a matter of personal preference. Cream or gel blushs literally melt into the skin and are easy to apply, while powder formulations can be dusted on quickly. Makeup artists advise that you should team your choice of blush with your foundation formulation: so, if you are wearing a creamy makeup base, go for cream blush, and if your foundation dries to a powdered finish, dust on powder blush.

SHADE SELECTION To find your most flattering shade of blush, pinch your cheeks, study the shade and try to match it with makeup. For a natural-looking finish, opt for a shade of blush that is one or two shades darker than your skin tone. If you go darker than this it will look unnatural. There is no need to invest in lots of different shades of blush; you can buy one color (such as a warm beige or soft brown) that will work with all makeup looks.

APPLICATION Always apply your blush after the rest of your makeup. Then you can add the right amount to balance your overall look. A quick and foolproof way is to smile when you brush on color to the cheek apples—that is, where you blush naturally. Use small circular motions to create a rosy-cheeked effect. Avoid enhancing the cheek apples if you have a particularly round face, as this will only accentuate the shape.

To softly sculpt the cheekbones, again apply blush in small circular motions, this time working down the cheekbone. This will prevent any unsightly stripes of color occurring. To give the skin on the cheeks a smooth, poreless finish, stroke blush downwards; if you go upwards, you run the risk of pushing pigment up and into your pores, thus highlighting any open ones. Always start applying color at the top of the cheeks and work down. This way, the color will gradually fade and you'll be left with the right amount of blush in the right places.

EXPERT ADVICE Add blush as the finishing touch to your makeup. The shade you wear does not have to match your lip and eye color but it should be from the same color family; otherwise it might disrupt the balance of the face. For example, wearing an orange blush with red lipstick is not flattering, unless you want to make a statement. A darker than usual shade of face powder can be used in place of blush. Face powders intended for black and Latina women are great choices as blushes for pale and medium-toned skin.

BLUSH MISHAPS If, having applied your blush, you find it looks too dark compared to the rest of your makeup, either buff it away with a velour powder puff and translucent powder or press a damp cosmetic sponge into the skin to lift off the color. To ensure the problem does not arise in the first place, apply cheek color lightly, remembering that it is better to build up color gradually than go for one heavy-handed application.

CUSTOMBLENDING

BLUSHING FACES
If your summer blush does not suit your paler winter face, dip the loaded blush brush into translucent powder before dusting on. Create your own blush by mixing a small amount of lipstick with face cream on the back of your hand and then dab on to the cheeks. Alternatively, dot a creamy lipstick on to the cheeks and gently blend into the skin.

IN THE MIX
You can mix existing products to create new colors and textures. To combine different lipsticks, either mix on the back of the hand using a lip brush or chop up the colors, place in a small dish and heat gently in the microwave for a couple of seconds, or until the lipsticks turn into a liquid. Pour into a palette and leave to set, before painting on with a brush.

POWDER PLAY
To blend loose face, eye or cheek powder, simply place in a bowl and mix together throroughly using a spatula. For a foolproof way to blend them, place in an airtight container with a lid and shake vigorously. Pressed powders are best mixed on the back of the hand, using your fingertips or a makeup brush, or crush them together with a palette knife.

PERFECT SHADE
Most brands sold in the U.S.—especially those found in drugstores—offer a wide array of color choices to accomodate different skin tones. But no matter what your coloring, few people have a perfectly uniform skin tone. You may need to invest in more than one foundation to find a complete match for every part of your face.

mix cosmetics to create new colors and textures

SHEER TINTS
If your makeup bag is full of brightly colored or extremely dark lip shades which you never wear, customize them with Vaseline. Prime the lips with Vaseline and then paint on lip color with a brush. This will make the darkest shades appear as a wash of color and is a great way to experiment with shades which you are not normally inspired to try.

POLISH WORK
To create new nail color combinations you can try layering different polishes. Apply intense, deeper colors as the base coat and then add a sheer or iridescent top coat. Great color combinations are red with gold, purple with silver, and fuchsia with iridescent ivory. Alternatively, try adding different colors to half-used bottles of polish and shake well to mix.

FOUNDATION FIXES
As the seasons change, your foundation requirements are likely to differ. In summer, if your foundation is too thick, dilute with moisturizer. In winter, if your foundation does not offer sufficient coverage, mix with a small amount of super-fine powder to thicken it. Alternatively, mix concealer and foundation together, then smooth on.

GLISTENING SKIN
Add a small amount of silver powder (crush a pressed eyeshadow, using the flat side of a ruler) to loose face powder. Blend together and dust on to shoulders or parts of the body that may be revealed when you are wearing cut-away clothing to give the skin luminosity. Alternatively, mix foundation containing light-reflecting particles with body moisturizer.

BEAUTY INTELLIGENCE

1 If your eyes need brightening, it is a good idea to use sheer, enlivening shades of creamy beige, iridescent pearl, soft lilac or sheer wine eye color.

2 If you don't have your concealer on hand, you can always use a brush dipped in foundation to cover any unsightly blemishes or under-eye circles.

3 Avoid using concealers that have either pink or orange undertones when attempting to cover blemishes. They will highlight rather than hide imperfections.

4 If you want your blush to look really natural once you have applied it, you need to choose a shade that mimics your skin color when you blush naturally.

5 If you want to look well groomed but not heavily made-up, ensure that you have no harsh makeup lines around the eyes. The secret is to blend thoroughly.

For blondes and those with fair hair, brown mascara is a more natural-looking option than black and if more definition is required a brown/black variety is suitable.

6

7

If you don't want to wear any makeup, try sweeping a large brush loaded with bronzing powder over your skin to create a healthy-looking golden finish.

If you want to wear a really pale shade of eyeshadow, try adding definition to the eyes with a pencil and mascara to avoid the chance of looking washed out.

8

9

The tone of your skin will change with the seasons, so adapt the color of your foundation to suit your face by diluting it with some oil-free moisturizer as needed.

You will get more mileage from your lipstick if you apply it with a lip brush. It is estimated that this way you can get at least twenty more applications.

10

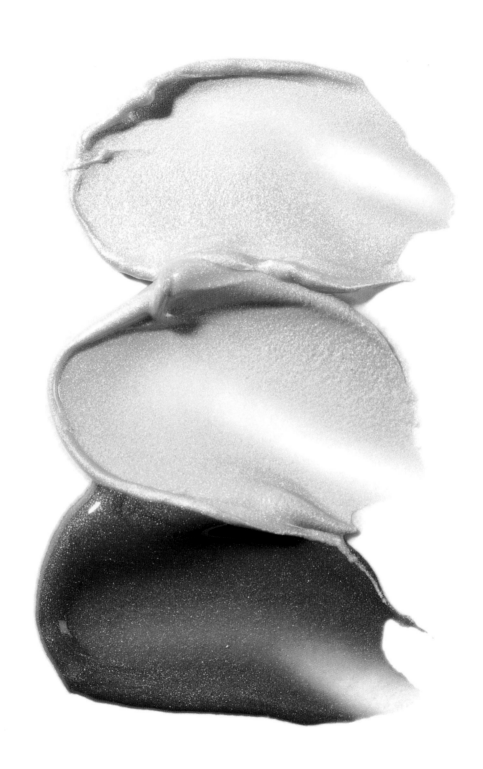

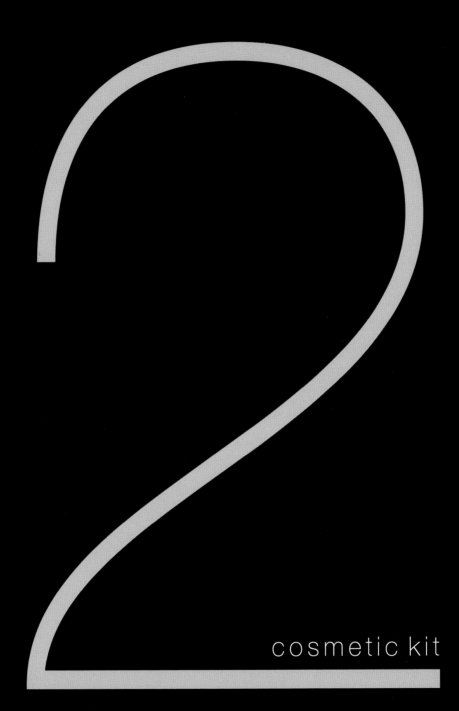

cosmetic kit

To achieve and maintain your best look, you don't need to be a beauty professional—or carry an enormous arsenal of makeup brushes. It is simply a matter of finding the tools of the trade that are most suited to your own particular beauty needs.

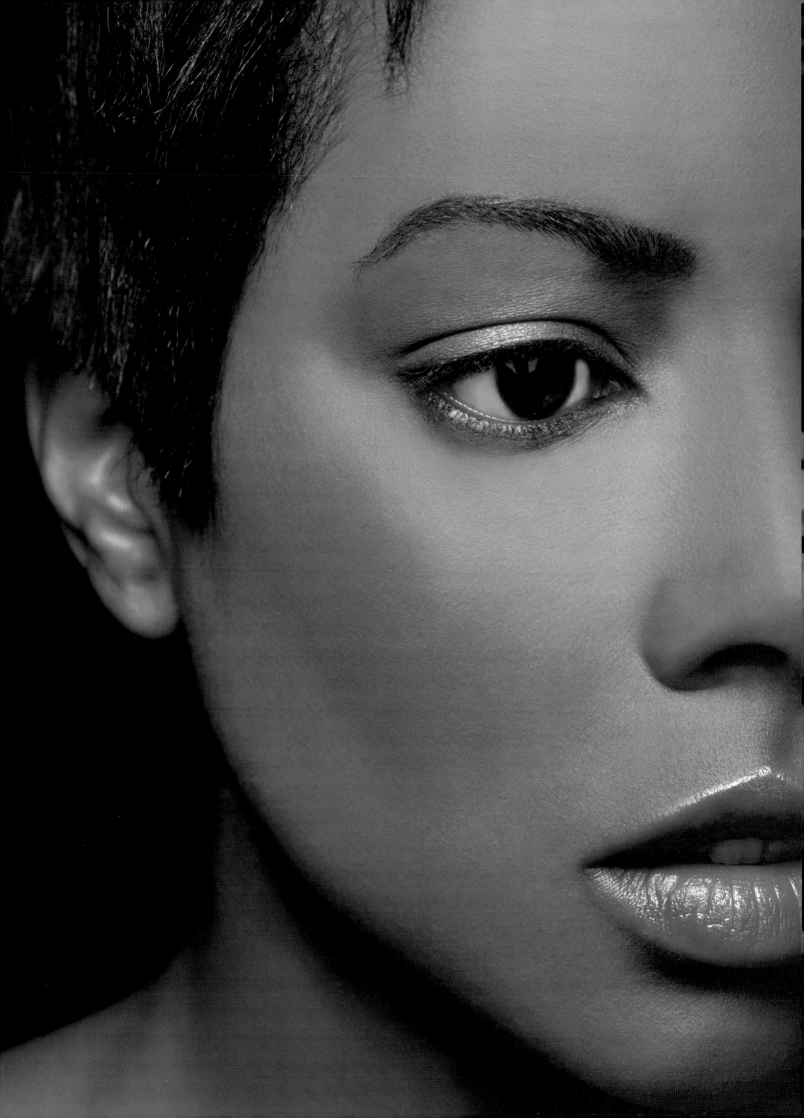

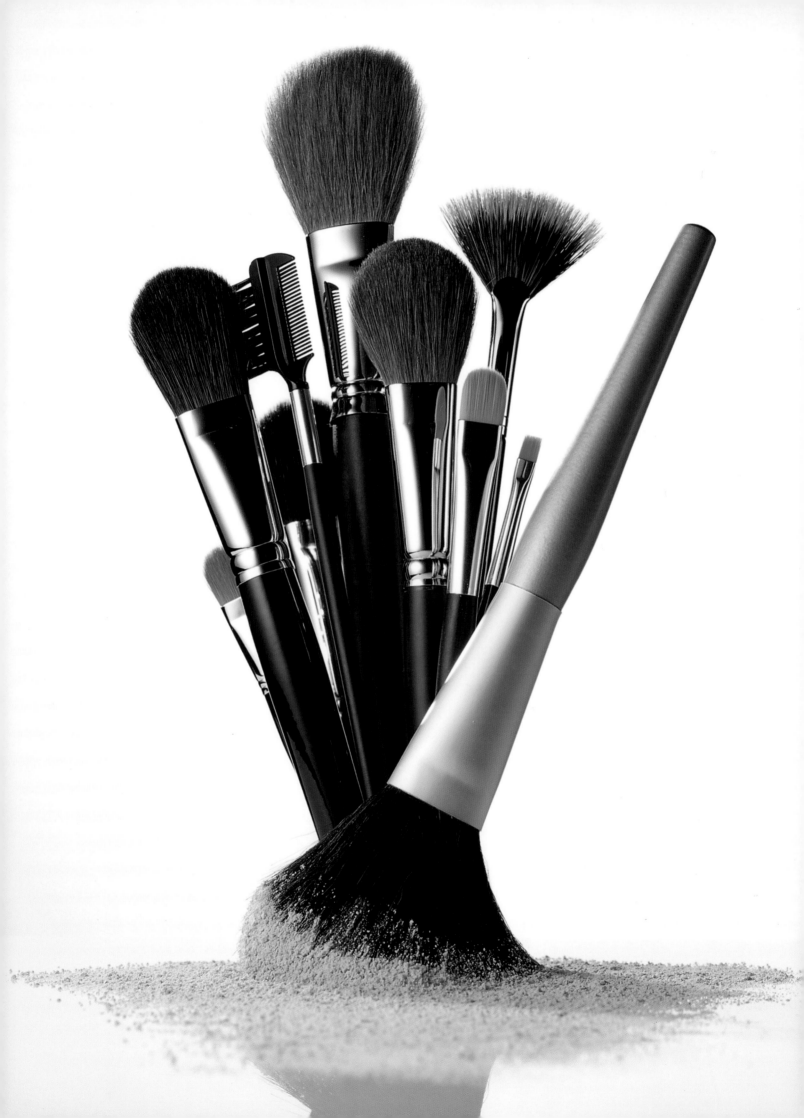

BRUSH BASICS

CHOOSING BRUSHES You don't need to arm yourself with every conceivable brush to perfect makeup application. In fact, you may prefer to apply some cosmetics with your fingertips or with the applicators provided. However, if you have trouble applying makeup, the right brushes can make all the difference. Knowing which ones to select and how to judge their quality can be daunting tasks. Makeup artists always advise investing in a set of good-quality brushes. Price usually gives some indication of quality, but when you're buying a brush you should also take into account how the bristles feel: too soft and they will not pick up and deposit color correctly; too prickly and they will irritate and possibly pierce the skin.

QUALITY CONTROL You can test the quality of a brush by running it over the back of your hand. If the bristles all move in the same direction, this is a good sign. However, if they splay on the skin, this indicates that the brush will offer little control, resulting in haphazard application. Also look at how the bristles shed. It is quite normal for new brushes to lose a few bristles, but if the loss is excessive this can indicate poor quality. Try gently pulling at the bristles: if more than a few come out in your hand, do not buy the brush. Make sure the handle of the brush feels comfortable to the touch and fits well in your hand. And think about the look you are hoping to achieve: brushes that are soft and do not have a lot of control are ideal for quick, easy application, while those that are compact and have much tighter bristles are ideal for precision application.

NATURAL VS SYNTHETIC There has been much debate over the years on the relative merits of using synthetic and real hair (the animals aren't made to suffer in any way in the process) for bristles in makeup brushes. The best-quality bristles come from goats, sables and blue squirrels, but synthetic bristles are much cheaper and can offer good results.

WHAT TO LOOK FOR To disguise pimples and imperfections with concealer, opt for a narrow brush with a flat, square tip. To apply powder, look for a soft-bristled, large brush which can be swept over the face in a couple of strokes. This can also be used to apply bronzing powder. To dust on powder blush, use brushes which are tapered at the sides and have a rounded tip; they have been designed specifically to contour and sculpt the cheekbones without leaving streaks of color. For filling sparse brows or shading and shaping the brows, look for a coarse-bristled brush that has a square or slant-edged tip. For applying eyeshadow, although sponge-tipped applicators are easy to control and make shading the eyelids a simple task, you could also use a soft-bristled brush with tapered sides and a rounded tip. This will help you create a more natural-looking, sheer finish than you'd achieve with a sponge-tipped applicator. For lining eyes with shadow, choose a small flat or angled brush with firm bristles. To shade and define the lips, look for a brush with firm tapered bristles.

EXPERT ADVICE Customize your makeup brushes to suit your needs. You can use scissors to taper the ends of brushes so they mold to your features. For example, you can give an eyeshadow brush a slant-edged finish so you can use it to line the eyes; or cut a coarse-bristled brush to a blunt finish and use it as a brow shader.

GROOMING TOOLS

TWEEZERS are an essential tool for keeping your brows neat. For plucking, choose a pair of long-handled, easy-to-hold ones with a slant edge to grip hairs effectively. For easing out ingrown hairs or splinters, go for tweezers with a fine point, but use them carefully as the sharp point can be dangerous.

SCISSORS should be a staple of any cosmetic kit for cutting nails and trimming unruly brows. Scissors with curved ends are suitable for shaping fingernails, while scissors with straight edges are good for cutting toenails and creating a square finish. To prolong their life, make sure you dry scissors thoroughly if they get wet and store them in a protective case.

PENCIL SHARPENERS don't have to be a costly investment. Art supply shops have inexpensive ones which work on most cosmetic pencils. Apart from keeping the points of liners and definers in shape, regular sharpening will help to ensure that they are clean and so prevent the spread of germs and bacteria.

COTTON SWABS are a must in your makeup kit in order to fix any number of problems that might arise, such as flaking mascara, smudged eyeliner or feathered lipstick.

MAKEUP SPONGES are not strictly necessary for applying foundation—you may prefer to smooth it on with your fingertips—but if you want to use a sponge, you should look for a triangular latex wedge or a natural sea sponge, which when dampened yields the sheerest application. These are available from beauty supply stores and are perfectly shaped to work around the nose or sweep under the eyes.

EYELASH CURLERS should have a place in any cosmetic kit as they will keep the lashes in good shape. When you curl your lashes, you will instantly appear more awake. Makeup artists recommend that you gently heat the ends of metal lash curlers with a hairdryer before using them to set the lashes in place. Just be careful not to burn the tender skin around the eyes.

POWDER PUFFS might not be vital but they do make applying powder a treat. Fluffy powder puffs feel great on the skin but they can overload the complexion with powder. For a more natural finish, makeup artists recommend using velour powder puffs to press powder into the skin, especially around the nose, on the chin and on the forehead—all areas that are prone to excessive shine.

BROW BRUSH & LASH COMB is a dual-purpose product that is handy for achieving a well-groomed finish even if you're not wearing makeup. A lash comb will help if your mascara clumps during application. Always plant the comb near the roots and gently move upwards as you drag it through the lashes to help define the natural curl. You can dip the edge of the brow brush in hair gel or moisturizer before running it through the brows to help keep them in place.

MAGNIFYING MIRRORS are helpful when plucking the eyebrows and checking that eyeliner is straight, imperfections are concealed and makeup is blended. Always place near natural light.

TISSUES are useful to have with you. They can be called upon to blot lipstick, to clean up overloaded mascara wands or, when pressed into the skin after the application of foundation, to absorb any excess oil from the product which will affect its staying power.

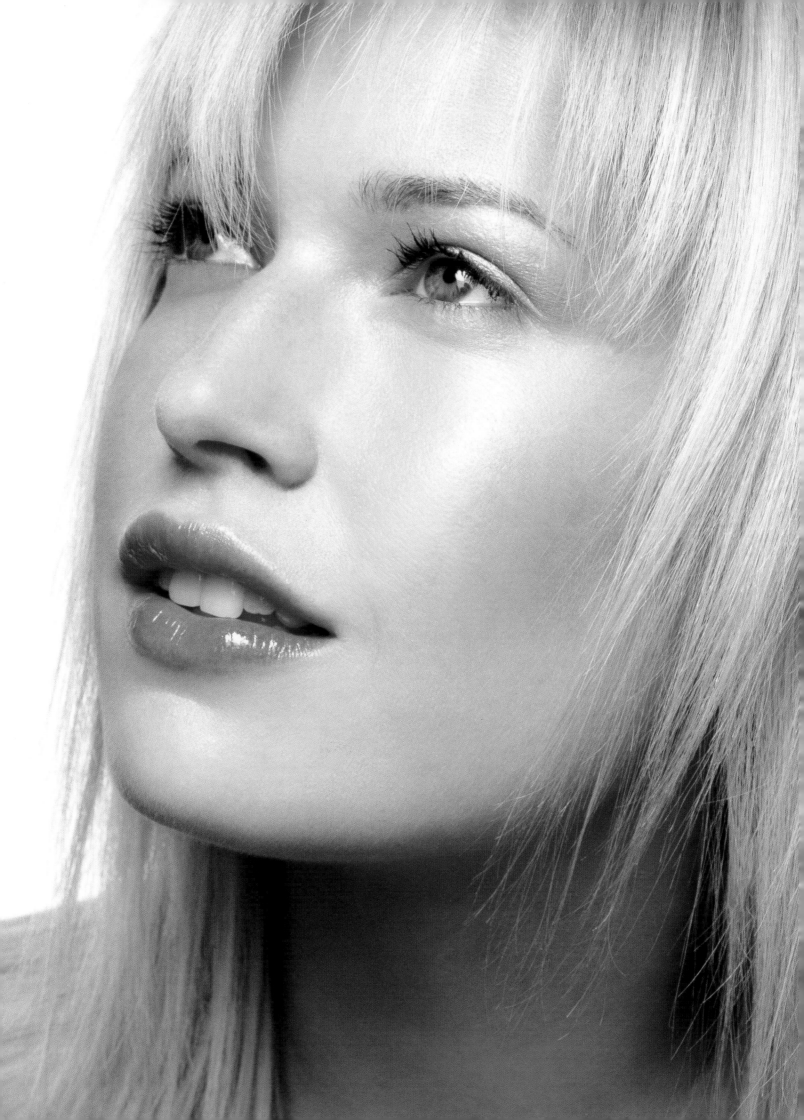

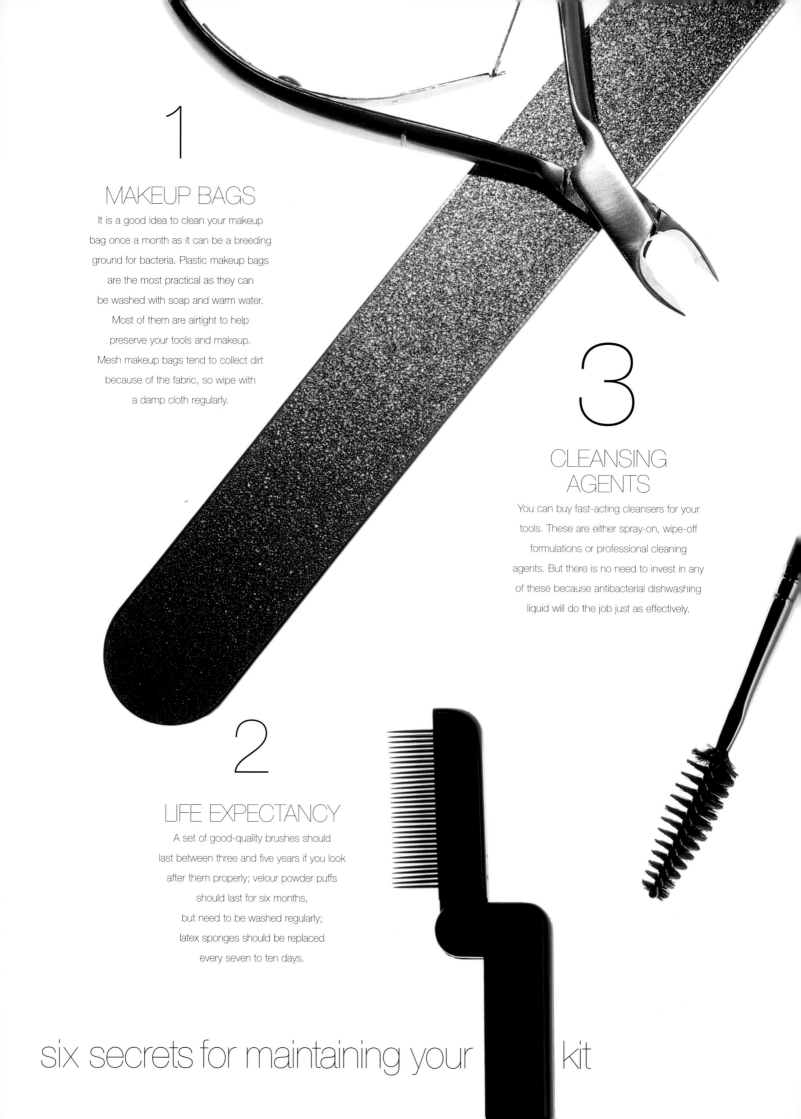

1
MAKEUP BAGS

It is a good idea to clean your makeup
bag once a month as it can be a breeding
ground for bacteria. Plastic makeup bags
are the most practical as they can
be washed with soap and warm water.
Most of them are airtight to help
preserve your tools and makeup.
Mesh makeup bags tend to collect dirt
because of the fabric, so wipe with
a damp cloth regularly.

3
CLEANSING AGENTS

You can buy fast-acting cleansers for your
tools. These are either spray-on, wipe-off
formulations or professional cleaning
agents. But there is no need to invest in any
of these because antibacterial dishwashing
liquid will do the job just as effectively.

2
LIFE EXPECTANCY

A set of good-quality brushes should
last between three and five years if you look
after them properly; velour powder puffs
should last for six months,
but need to be washed regularly;
latex sponges should be replaced
every seven to ten days.

six secrets for maintaining your kit

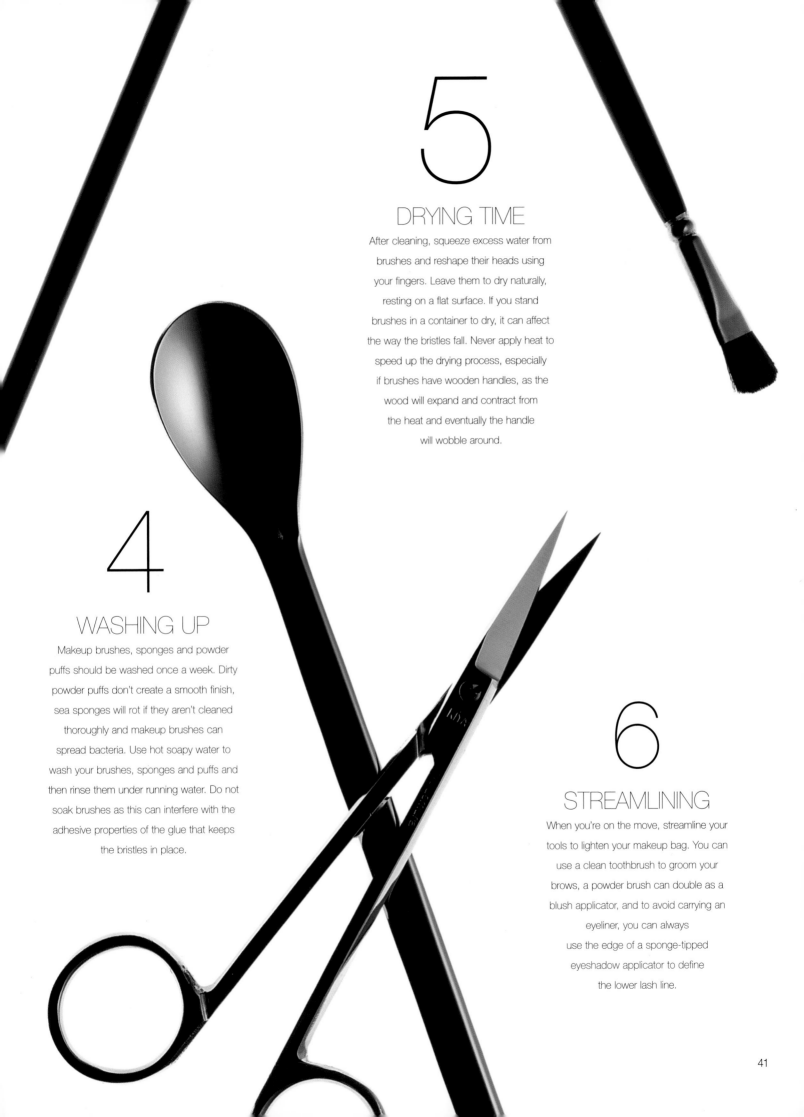

5

DRYING TIME

After cleaning, squeeze excess water from brushes and reshape their heads using your fingers. Leave them to dry naturally, resting on a flat surface. If you stand brushes in a container to dry, it can affect the way the bristles fall. Never apply heat to speed up the drying process, especially if brushes have wooden handles, as the wood will expand and contract from the heat and eventually the handle will wobble around.

4

WASHING UP

Makeup brushes, sponges and powder puffs should be washed once a week. Dirty powder puffs don't create a smooth finish, sea sponges will rot if they aren't cleaned thoroughly and makeup brushes can spread bacteria. Use hot soapy water to wash your brushes, sponges and puffs and then rinse them under running water. Do not soak brushes as this can interfere with the adhesive properties of the glue that keeps the bristles in place.

6

STREAMLINING

When you're on the move, streamline your tools to lighten your makeup bag. You can use a clean toothbrush to groom your brows, a powder brush can double as a blush applicator, and to avoid carrying an eyeliner, you can always use the edge of a sponge-tipped eyeshadow applicator to define the lower lash line.

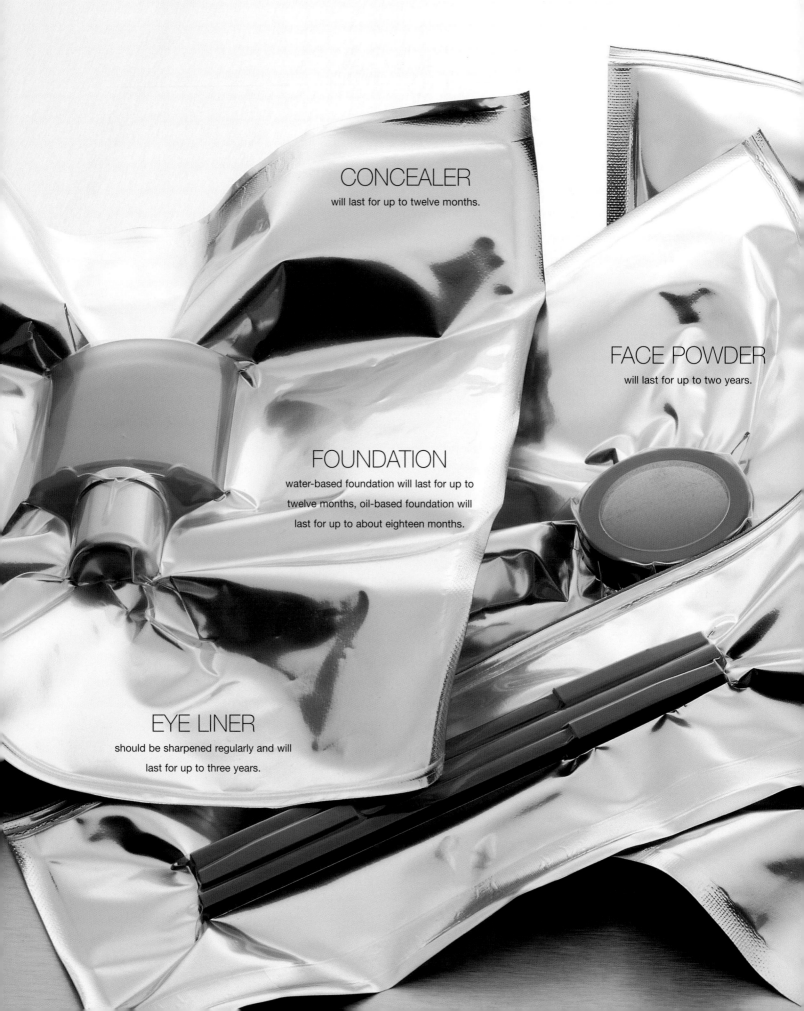

SHELF LIFE

CONCEALER

will last for up to twelve months.

FACE POWDER

will last for up to two years.

FOUNDATION

water-based foundation will last for up to
twelve months, oil-based foundation will
last for up to about eighteen months.

EYE LINER

should be sharpened regularly and will
last for up to three years.

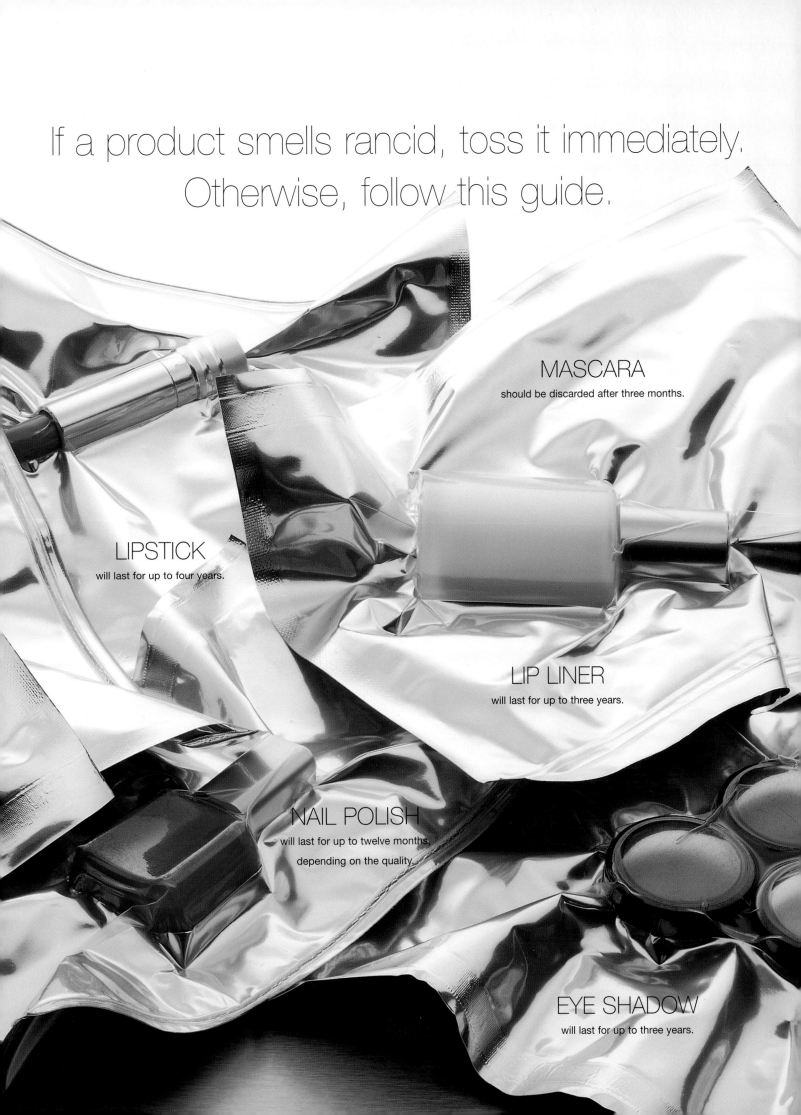

SEASONALCHANGES

FOUNDATION

During the winter months opt for a creamy foundation that helps prevent skin from dehydrating, and when the heat is on during the summer months switch to an oil-free formulation. The skin produces more oil during the hot weather and so these formulations will work with the skin's natural balance. Lightweight, tinted moisturizers are also a good option.

POWDER

Pressed or loose powder can be used year-round, but an oil-free formula is a better choice in summer when skin is oilier, as an oil-free powder is less likely to clog your pores. If you want a healthy glow, replace your face powder with bronzing powder during the summer. Look for a bronzer that is laced with subtle shimmer to make your skin look luminous as well as healthy.

BLUSH

Creamy formulations will melt into the skin and won't have a drying effect, making them ideal for winter wear; powder blush can be a good option for the summer as it helps absorb surface oils. Try wearing lavender pink shades to brighten the pallor of winter complexions; in the summer, choose soft peaches and burnished browns to warm the skin.

BASE

If you smooth on foundation only to find it looks slightly too dark for your skin tone, instead of removing and starting again, simply press translucent face powder into the skin to tone down the color. Afterwards, if your skin looks too powdery, spray with a fine mist of water.

adapt your makeup bag to suit the season

COLOR
Although there are no strict rules about what you can and cannot wear, try to adapt your color palette to suit the season. During the winter, if you look sallow or washed-out, warm up your skin with brighter makeup shades like peach, tawny pink and bronze. During the summer, copper, burnished browns and golds are flattering to all skin tones.

FORMULATIONS
During the summer, it is best to steer clear of makeup products that are creamy and prone to melt and slide off your skin. When it's hot, cheeks will be naturally rosy, so you could skip blush. If your mascara tends to flake and smudge in the heat, you might consider having your lashes tinted. Just be sure to go to a reputable salon.

MASCARA
Mascara is a trans-seasonal item, so the only change you may wish to make to substitute your existing mascara with a waterproof one during the summer months or when you go on vacation. Waterproof formulations can be drying on the lashes, so coat them with a thin film of Vaseline as a conditioning treat at night, once every two weeks or when your lashes feel brittle.

LIPSTICK
For winter wear, look for a moisture-rich lipstick that will help protect the lips from chapping and dryness. Avoid wearing lipsticks that dry to a matte finish as they can have a dehydrating effect. During the summer, look for a lipstick with sunscreen to help protect against the sun's harmful UV rays. Sheer tints and lip glosses are ideal for summer wear.

BEAUTY INTELLIGENCE

1

Before tweezing your brows, cleanse your skin. If you cannot stand the pain of plucking, numb the area first with babies' teething gel.

2

If your nail scissors are blunt or the edges of your tweezers have lost their grip, you can run sandpaper gently over the inner blunt edges to sharpen them.

3

Don't try to salvage nail polish that has dried out by diluting it with nail polish remover. It will not solve the problem, so just throw it away.

4

When you're looking for makeup brushes, try art supply stores. You can pick up great brushes at reasonable prices.

5

Try not to lend makeup brushes to other people as this can spread their oils onto your skin. If someone does borrow your brushes, wash them thoroughly before reusing.

When the bristles of your brushes start to become messy and begin to fray, revamp them by using a pair of nail scissors to trim stray hairs back into shape.

6 After applying your moisturizer, you should always allow the skin to absorb it for at least ten minutes before smoothing any makeup on top.

7 You should never buff your nails after taking a bath or shower, because they'll be too soft and damage might occur to the surrounding skin.

8 To ensure that your tweezers maintain their firm grip, regularly wipe the tips with rubbing alcohol to remove any oily buildup that might have settled.

9 Your fingers are great applicators too. Because they will absorb some of the makeup's color, they're best for a sheer, light finish.

10

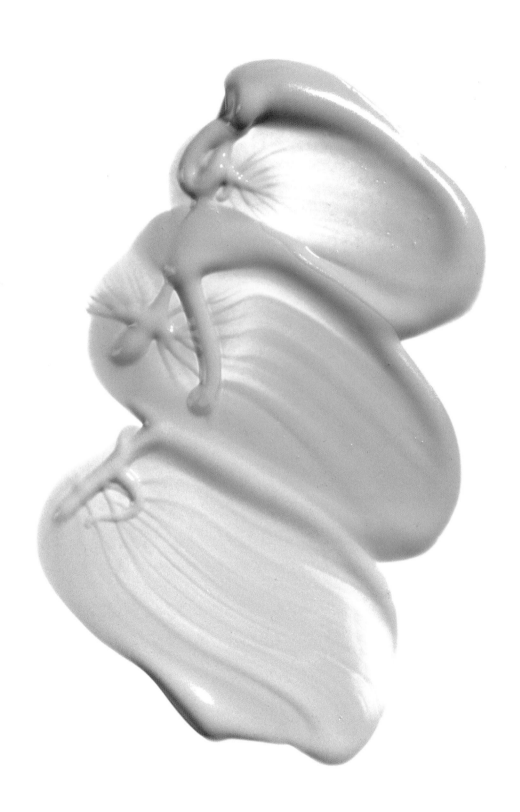

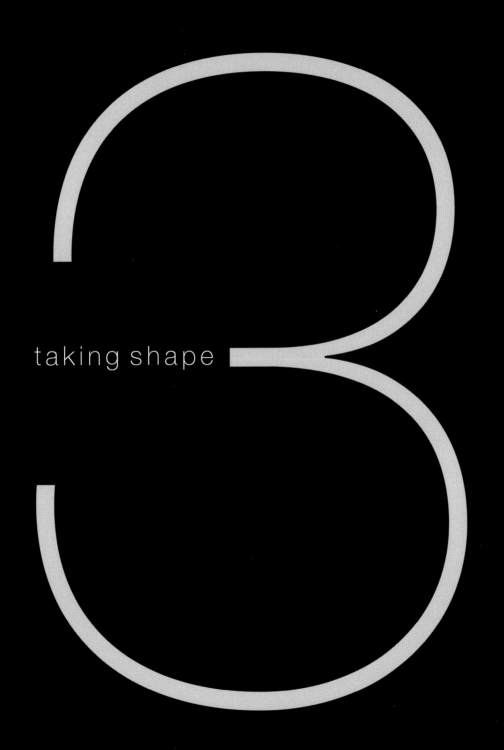

taking shape

In your ideal world maybe you imagine yourself genetically blessed with model-like looks, but the reality is that most of us have features which are not perfect. You may worry about having a prominent nose, small, deep-set eyes or uneven lips, but these are actually what give your face its individuality, so try treating them as marks of beauty.

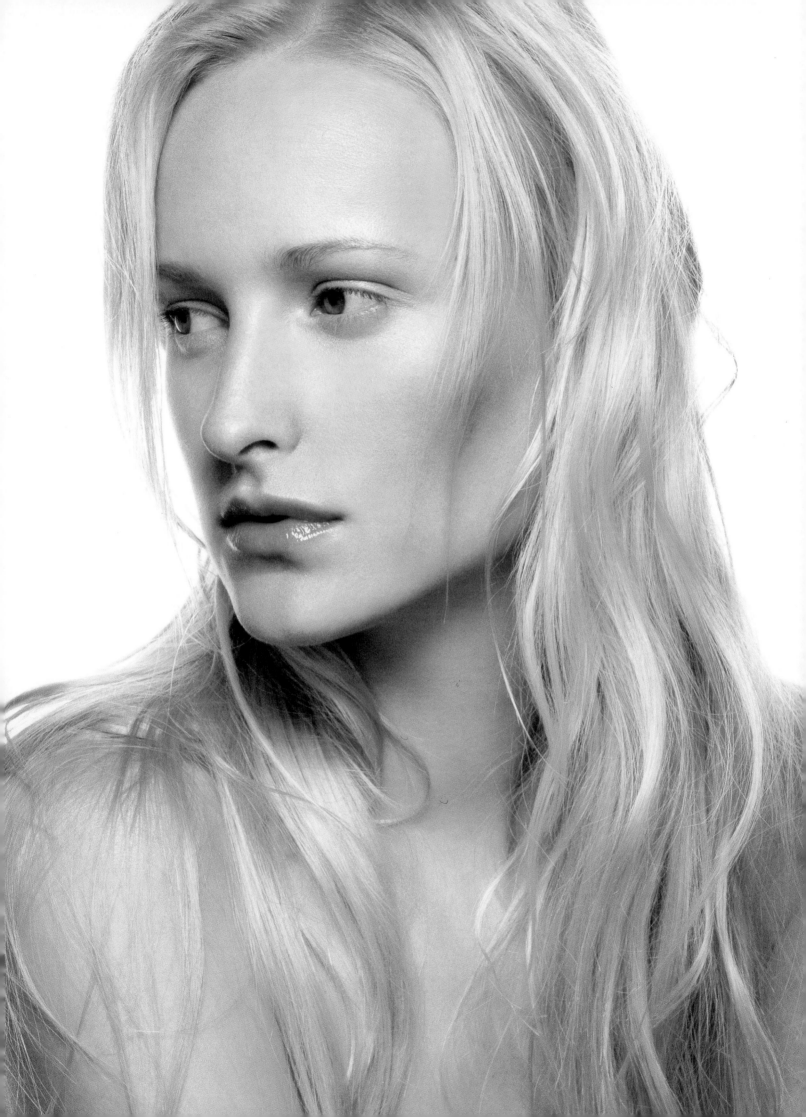

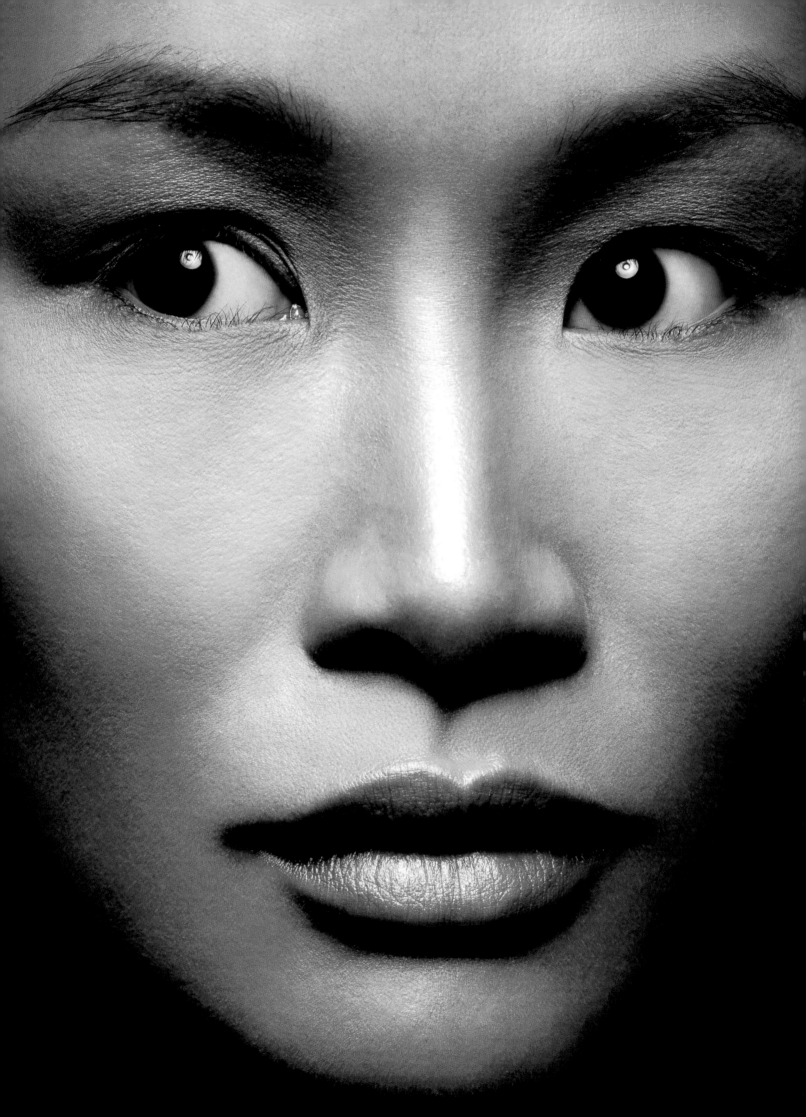

CHEEKBONES

If you don't have prominent cheekbones, you can create them with makeup. Look for a face powder or blush that matches the natural shadows created under your cheekbones. To get the contour in the correct place, gently suck in your cheeks and then apply color right beneath the cheekbones.

ROUND FACE

Round faces, which are usually short and fairly wide with full cheeks and a rounded chin, have the advantage of always looking youthful. To make the most of your face, avoid accentuating the shape. Do not wear blush on the apples of your cheeks, but instead softly sculpt the cheekbones. Avoid the kohl-rimmed look. Apply eye shadow and liner in such a way that they elongate the eyes and balance the face. Your brow should be tapered toward the tip of the ear. If you wear glasses, slim down your face with square, rectangular or cat's-eye frames.

ELONGATED FACE

Elongated faces usually have high cheekbones, a high forehead and a chiselled jawline. To balance an elongated face, do not make the arch of the eyebrow too extreme; rather, soften your features and keep your brow shape in a straight line that tapers toward the tip of the ear. Apply blush to the apples of your cheeks in small circular motions to create a rosy-faced effect. If you wear glasses, look for frames that are round or curved, because these will help break up the narrow shape of your face.

HEART-SHAPED FACE

Wider around the forehead and curving down to a point, this kind of face shape can look very dainty and pretty. To enhance the overall shape, highlight the tip of the chin using a face powder or highlighter that suits your skin tone. Work on the temples next, blending the color into the hairline (you will need to be careful if you have blonde hair because the color will show). Add blush to the cheek hollows (the areas just below the cheekbone). If you have small features, play up your lips or eyes with color to give your face increased definition.

SQUARE FACE

Square faces tend to feature a broad forehead and jaw. To soften the strong angles of this shape, dust a face powder one shade darker than what you'd normally wear around the hair- and jawline. Apply blush to the apples of your cheeks in small, circular motions. When grooming the brows, ensure that their ends curve toward the middle of the ear. If you wear glasses, look for thin frames in oval or round shapes as they will balance your face.

MOLES & FRECKLES

If you have a mole on your face, make it your signature. Makeup artists transform moles (or large freckles) into beauty spots with waterproof eye liners. Simply shade the area with a black pencil. But if you notice any changes in color, appearance or texture of your mole, see a dermatologist immediately. Do not pluck hairs from moles; simply trim with nail scissors. Freckles and brown spots can be treated with a fade cream that contains hydroquinone or licorice extract.

TOOTH TACTICS

If your teeth aren't perfect, wearing brightly colored or strong shades of lipstick can draw attention to the mouth. If your tooth enamel is stained despite twice-yearly professional cleanings—which can occur from the tannin in tea, the caffeine in drinks, eating certain foods and smoking—try commercially available tooth-whitening pastes, strips or kits. Avoid frosted peach and creamy beige tones of lipstick, as these have a tendency to make your teeth appear more yellow.

DOUBLE CHIN

To make a double chin less obvious, use face powder one shade darker than normal to softly shade the chin area. This will create the illusion that your chin is receding. Dab highlighter on the tip of the chin to brighten it. Make sure you blend thoroughly for a natural-looking finish.

FACIAL HAIR

Excessive facial hair can either be a hereditary condition or the result of a hormone imbalance. If the condition is severe, contact your doctor and have a blood test to detect imbalances and receive treatment. There are three main ways to deal with facial hair: waxing, which removes hairs for up to six weeks; electrolysis, which uses a needle to target each hair individually, zapping it at the roots (the drawback is that a course of treatments is required to permanently remove them all); and laser treatment, which targets hair at the roots with nearly immediate results, although maintenance sessions are required. Bleaching is a less-costly at-home alternative.

PROMINENT NOSE

If you have a prominent nose and are self-conscious about it, wear a strong lip color or make your eyes the focal point of your face with makeup, thus drawing attention away from the nose. To soften and streamline the bridge of the nose, dust on a pressed powder one shade lighter than your skin tone, working down either side of the bridge of your nose and then up toward the eyebrows.

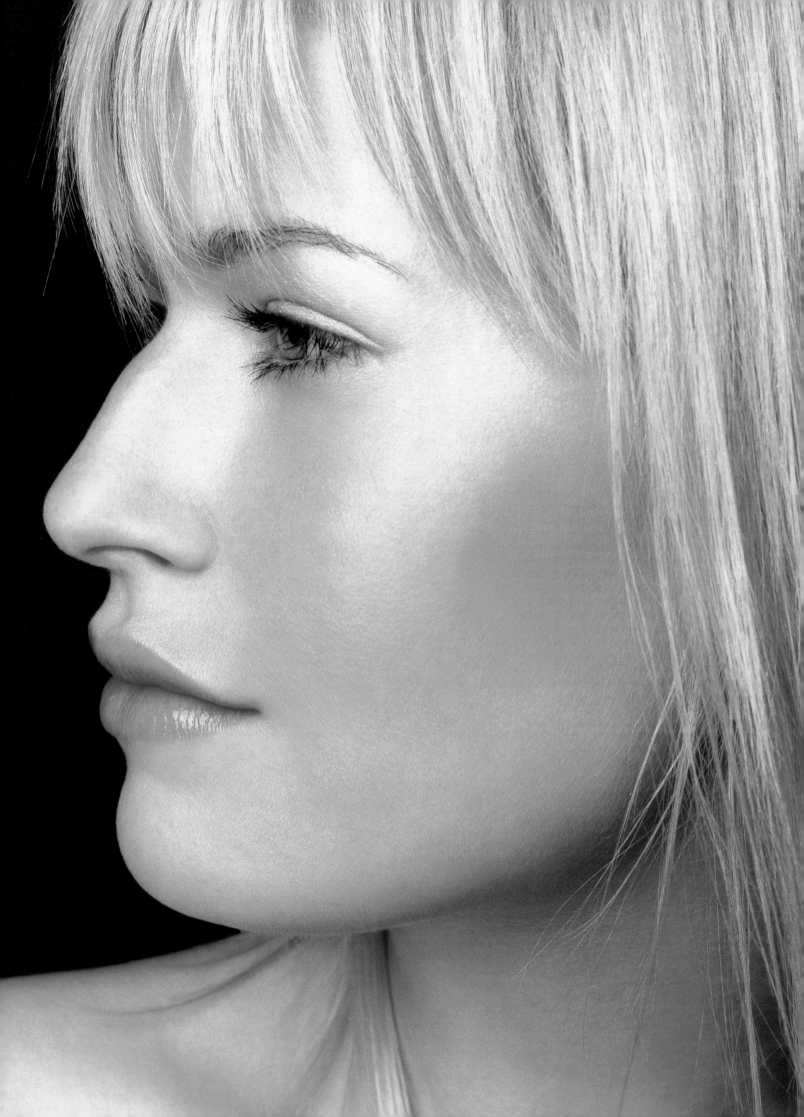

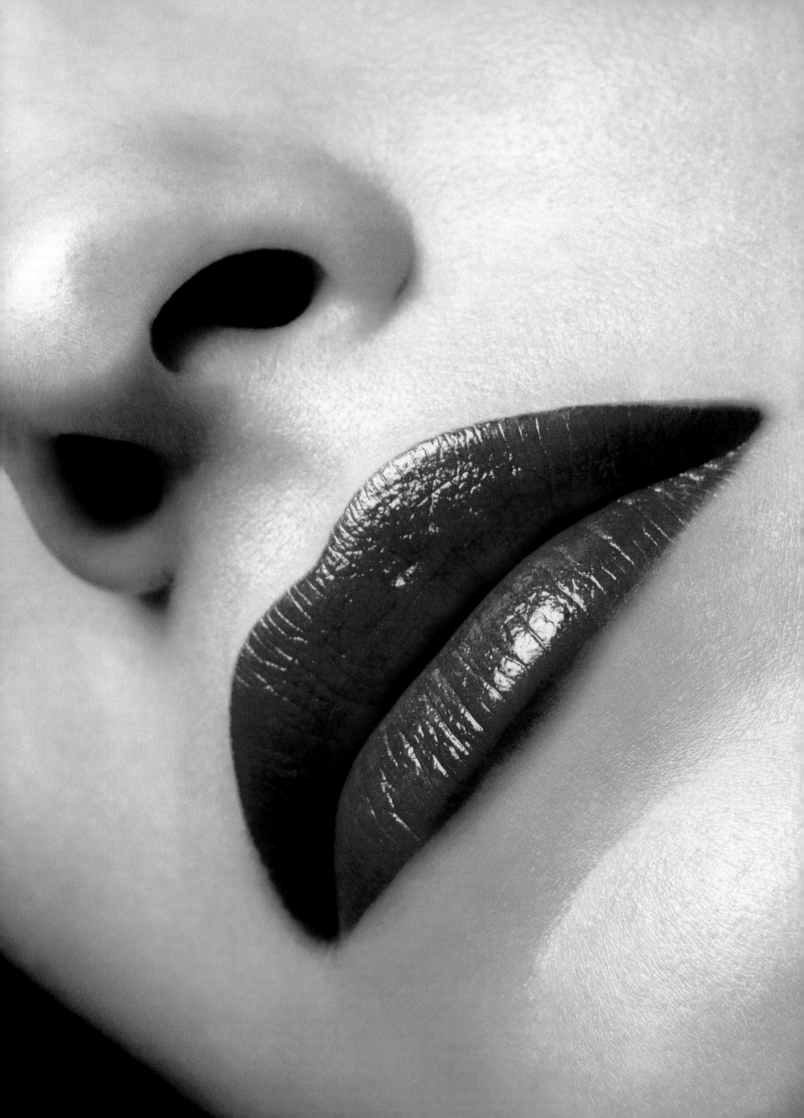

LIP SHAPES

THIN LIPS There is no point trying to draw a line outside your natural lip line in an attempt to make your lips appear bigger. It will just look messy and unnatural. Instead, to create the illusion of fullness, wear light- to medium-toned lipsticks or glosses. Concentrate the color in the center of your mouth, then blend out. Avoid wearing bright reds or very dark lip colors with matte finishes because they can give thin lips a drawn appearance.

FULL LIPS If you have full, luscious lips, make the most of them and paint on a bold shade of lipstick—remember, many women pay good money to have their lips plumped up with collagen injections! However, for those who want to play down fullness, skip lip liner and wear paler shades of lipstick. Avoid gloss, as it only accentuates fullness; matte is a better option. To draw attention away from the lips, wear only a hint of lip color and instead, play up your eyes.

UNEVEN LIPS It is very common to have a thinner top lip and fuller bottom lip—this is true for over 90 percent of women. To achieve better balance, outline the outside edge of the top lip, and keep within the natural shape of the lower lip. If the disparity really bothers you, try using a lighter shade of lipstick on the upper lip and then a slightly darker shade of the same color on the bottom lip. Purse the lips together after application. This should create a more even look. If in your case the bottom lip is thinner than the top one, reverse the techniques just described.

BROAD LIPS To draw attention away from the width of the lips, use liner to emphasize your Cupid's bow, thus adding extra height to the upper lip. After applying color, dab silver gloss onto the center of the lower lip, over your lipstick. Apart from creating an interesting finish, this will direct attention to the center of your mouth and away from the edges of your lips.

LITTLE LIPS Medium-toned lipsticks will look very attractive on small lips, whereas dark, strong shades are not as flattering. Experiment with a range of different textures to make the most of small lips, looking especially for shimmery, glossy or sheer tints in brighter colors. To accentuate lips, after applying your lipstick, use lip pencil in a color that is slightly darker than the lipstick to shade the outer sections of the upper and lower lips. Blend in with your lipstick using your fingertip or a makeup brush. This will give your lips improved definition, which in turn will create the illusion that they are bigger than they really are.

DOWN-TURNED LIPS You can lift a down-turned mouth by applying concealer around the outer edges of the lips, since this is where a natural shadow may be cast. This will instantly highlight the area and lift the mouth. Do not apply dark colors, especially around the outer corners of the lips, and do not use lip liner to trace the natural contour of the lips, both of which will only accentuate droopiness. Opt instead for paler shades, focusing the intensity of the color on the central part of your mouth. Go for sheer textures to get the very best results.

EYE SHAPES

SMALL EYES This shape is characterized by a short distance between the upper and lower lashes. To visually open up the eyes, experiment with light shades of eyeshadow. Avoid dark colors as they will make the eyes appear even smaller. Sweep a wash of color in a light shade over the eyelid to enlarge and illuminate the eyes, then shade the outer corner of the lid and the crease with a slightly darker shade. Define the outer corners of the upper and lower eye with a pencil, tapering the line outwards to elongate the eyes. Then, add a subtle highlight to the top of the brow bone and apply lots of mascara. Keep your brows well groomed to ensure that there are no stray hairs on the brow area, as this can enclose the eye.

WIDE-SET To make your eyes appear closer together, focus shadow and liner on the inner corners of the eyes. Start by sweeping a light shadow over the whole eye area, then dust a medium color onto the inner half of the eyelid and blend outward to create a natural finish. Next, line from the inner corner to the middle of the eye and then blend outward. Last, coat your lashes with mascara.

CLOSE-SET If your eyes are less than one eye-length apart, create the illusion of added width by keeping the inner corners of the eyes light and bright and then shading the outer corners. Sweep a light shadow across the eyelid, then dust a medium shade onto the outer half of the eyelid. With eyeliner, define from the middle of the top and bottom lash line, extending and tapering the line up and out, a little past the outer corner of the eyes. Concentrate mascara on the outermost lashes.

DEEP-SET If you have deep-set eyes, your brow bone will be more prominent than your eyelid, so you'll want to make the eyelid more pronounced and create a balance between the upper and lower lids. Use a light- to medium-toned shadow over the entire eyelid, then a slightly darker shade above the eye crease to play down the brow bone. Define the upper lash line with a pencil, keeping the line fine on the inner corner of the eyes and thicker on the middle of the eyelid, then tapering it out. Repeat on the lower lash line, smudging for a natural effect. Highlight the brow bone and add several coats of your favorite mascara.

ASIAN EYES The eyelids of Asian women are sometimes invisible when the eyes are open, so for definition sweep a medium-toned eyeshadow over the eyelid and brow area. Dust under the brow with pale highlighter to bring out the brow bone and add contrast to the eyes. Use a pencil eyeliner, keeping the line very fine and natural-looking along upper and lower lash lines. Or, instead of eyeshadow, paint on a thick smoky line along the upper lash line and under the eye.

DROOPY EYES Down-turned eyes can be lifted—with makeup! Keep the attention on the eyelids rather than the lash lines. Apply eyeshadow to the outer corner of the eyelid, extending the color up and out in a feline shape. Add highlighter to the brow bone using a very light shade. Avoid using eyeliner as it will trace the droopy contour. Use mascara, concentrating on the lashes at the inner corner of the eyes—this will have a "lifting" effect. Or, try a smudge of silver shadow on the inner corners of the eyes to brighten and, again, to lift.

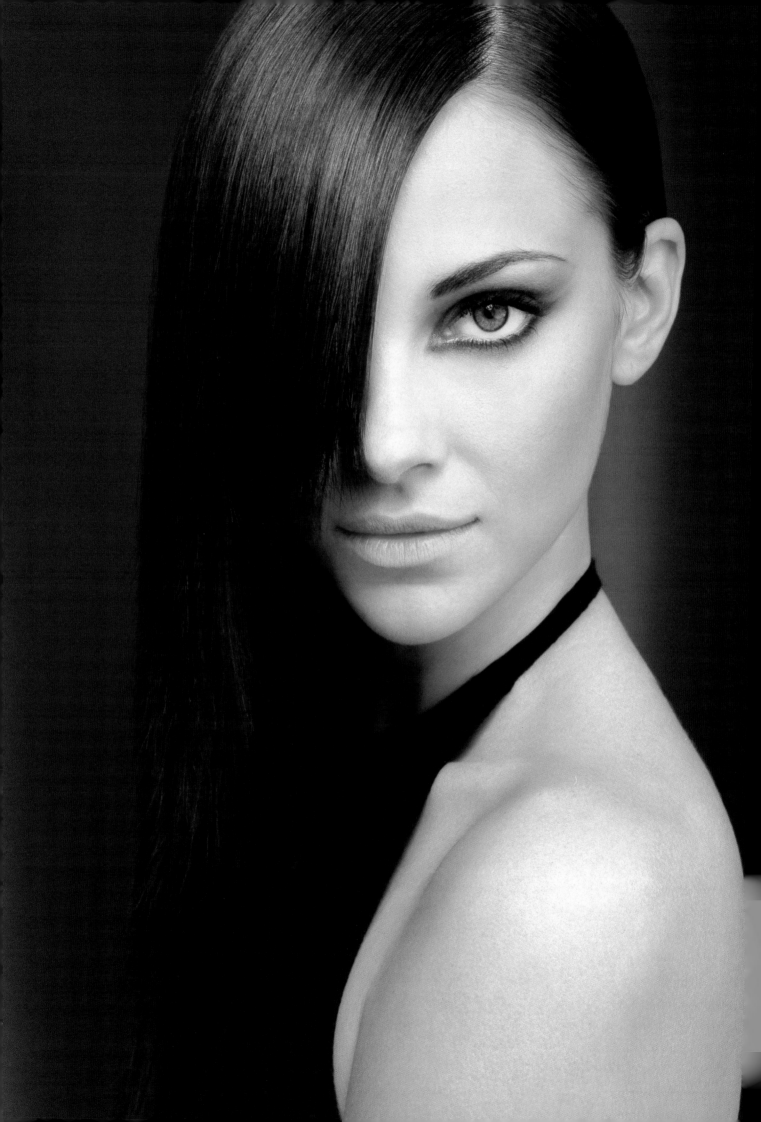

FOUNDATION

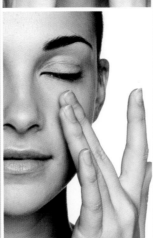

1. Apply compact foundation with a sponge; apply liquid formulas with your fingertips, a foundation brush, or a sponge. There is no need to whitewash the complexion with foundation. You should simply dab it on where it is really needed, such as areas of uneven skin tone, open pores and broken blood vessels.

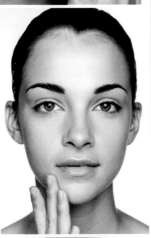

2. Ensure that coverage is even and blend foundation thoroughly. Work over the jawline and down the neck, so it's not obvious where your foundation starts and finishes.

3. Using a brush or your fingertips, dab concealer under the eyes and then disguise any imperfections. To cover pimples, apply the concealer with a small brush, concentrating on the center of the blemish and then feathering slowly outward.

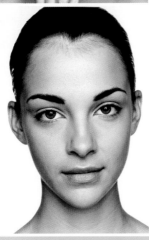

4. After applying foundation, blot your face with a tissue to remove any excess oil in the product, which can interfere with the staying power of your base. Check your work in natural daylight.

POWDER

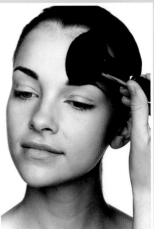

1. Use loose or pressed powder to set your foundation. Always dust powder onto the skin in downward strokes, as this prevents particles of powder from getting trapped under your facial hairs and creates an even finish.

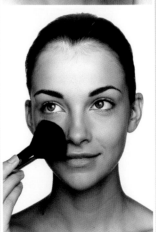

2. You do not need to apply powder all over the face. Concentrate on areas prone to shine, such as the nose, the chin and the forehead. Apply sparingly and aim to give your skin a seemingly unmade-up finish.

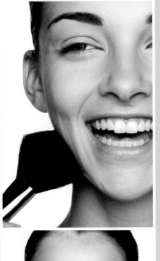

3. When retouching, blot the skin with a tissue and then dust on face powder. This will remove any build-up of product, which combined with the skin's natural oils will produce an unflattering finish.

4. Finally, when you have applied your powder, spray your face with a fine mist of water. Gently press a tissue onto the face with your fingertips and then smoothly lift it off. This will guarantee you are left with a natural-looking finish that is not too powdery or dull.

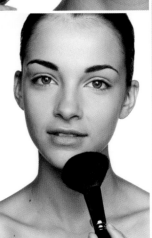

EYESHADOW

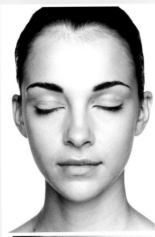

1. The simplest and most effective way to define the eyes is to use what is known as the three-step method of application. Select three eyeshadows in different shades from the same color family: for example, a pale ivory, a medium terracotta and a deep bronze.

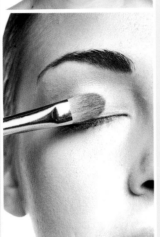

2. Use the lightest shade to color the eyelid. Work outward from the inner corner of the lid. Do not take the color right up into the crease, but rather apply it in small sweeping strokes all over the eyelid.

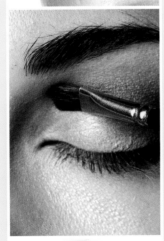

3. Next, using the medium-tone eyeshadow, shade the crease, working out from the inner corner. Try raising your eyebrows to gently lift the eyes, as this should make it easier for you to define the line.

4. Finish by using the palest shade to add a touch of color to the brow bone. Check your work in natural daylight. If further blending is required, use your fingertips or work over the eye with a small, clean makeup brush.

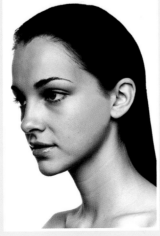

BROW DEFINERS

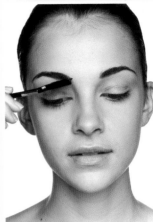

1. Defining the eyebrows helps to frame the face. Before defining, brush through brows with a brow comb to remove any stray hairs or particles of foundation and face powder. Brush through first in the opposite direction of the natural hair growth, then rebrush into shape.

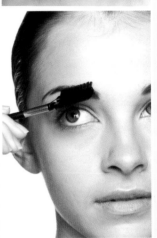

2. Use a brow definer (either a pencil or powder) in a shade that that matches your natural brow color. When defining with a pencil, apply in small feathered strokes (no longer than the average length of a brow hair). Whether you're using a pencil or powder, start at the inner corner of the brow and gradually taper outward for the best results.

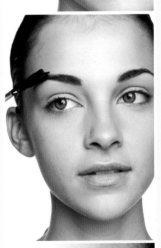

3. Then carefully rub the brows with a brush or your fingertip to ensure they don't look too heavily made up. If you've been heavy-handed, use a moist cotton swab to gently roll over the brow to lift off any excess color.

4. Last, brush your brows back into place. Brow gel helps your brows keep their shape all day long.

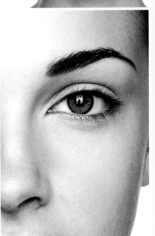

MASCARA

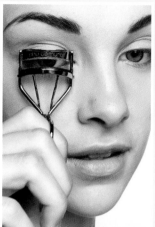

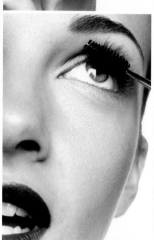

1. To give your lashes the best definition possible, use an eyelash curler before applying mascara. Wipe the mascara wand first with a tissue to remove any excess product.

2. Then plant the wand into the eyelashes, close to the roots, and slowly pull through, while gently working the brush back and forth in a zig-zag motion. As well as applying the mascara, this will also help reinforce the curl.

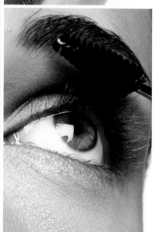

3. Work through the eyelashes with a lash comb to separate and define. Make sure that the fine wispy lashes on the outer corners of the eyes have picked up sufficient mascara. If they haven't, use the tip of the wand to define these stragglers.

4. Once the first coat of mascara is dry (this will take about sixty seconds), apply a second coat. Two fine coats will always look much more professional than one heavy-handed application. Finally, once both coats are dry, brush through again with a lash comb if required.

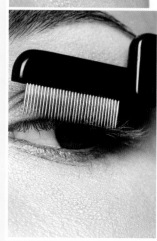

LIP LINERS

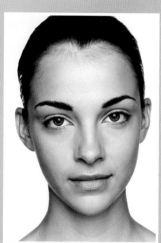

1. To ensure staying power, prime your lips with foundation before applying lip liner. Look for an oil-free or a long-lasting formula. Or, choose a long-wearing lip liner. If your lips are prone to dryness, try coating them with a thin film of non-greasy lip balm first.

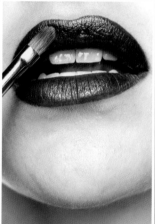

2. Do not attempt to draw one unbroken line around the lips. Unless you are a real professional, the chances are that your line will be uneven, and will also look dated and unnatural. Instead, for the best results, try applying the liner in small feathered strokes around the lips.

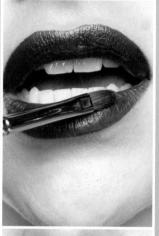

3. Then work over the entire lip area with lip liner, shading the lower and upper lips. Choose a shade similar to your natural lip color or one to complement your choice of lipstick.

4. Finish by blending with a lip brush so as not to leave any harsh lines. If you don't want to wear lipstick as a top coat, slick on lip gloss instead.

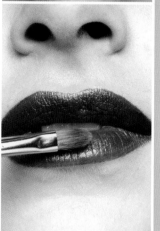

LIPSTICK

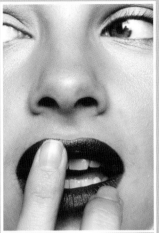

1. Ideally, you should apply lipstick with a brush. Start at the outer corners of the lower lip and then fill in the central area. Once you are satisfied with the results, repeat this process on the upper lip. Finish by blotting your lips gently with a tissue to remove any excess product.

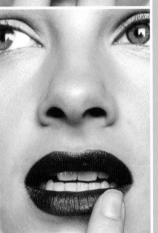

2. Reapply lipstick and then repeat the process of blotting with a tissue and coating with lipstick several times. If you want to make extra sure that your lipstick will stay put, apply pressed powder to your lips between coats.

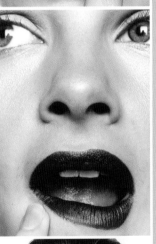

3. For a more dramatic look, dab a bright lip color that corresponds to your base shade onto the center of the upper and lower lips, (think tone-on-tone) then purse the lips together. You'll find this will create a wearable, "bee-stung" look.

4. Add the finishing touches by dabbing lip gloss on to the center of the lower lip. This will create the illusion of fuller lips.

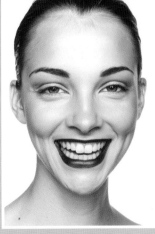

BLUSH

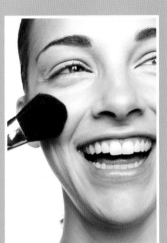

1. Before you apply your powder blush, blow on the brush to remove any excess product. If you overdo your blush, you can tone down the color by dusting with translucent powder or blotting with a damp makeup sponge.

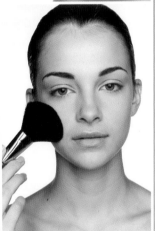

2. To softly sculpt the cheekbones, apply your blush in small circular motions, working carefully down the cheekbone. This will ensure that you are left with a natural-looking finish instead of unsightly stripes of color.

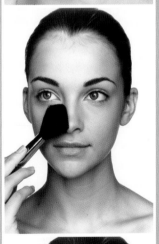

3. In order to define the apples of your cheeks, locate the cheekbone and dab on color just below. Massage it into the skin, again working in small circular motions. This will give your skin a healthy flush of color.

4. If you would like to add a flattering highlight to your cheeks, use your fingertips to dab a shimmering highlighter onto the top of the cheekbone. Working away from the eyes, blend downward. You want to create a soft, subtle effect, so try to apply the highlighter sparingly.

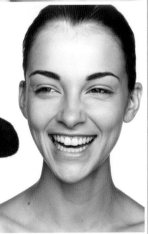

CORRECTIONWORK

SHADOW FIX

If your choice of eyeshadow looks wrong, you can lift off the color without messing up the rest of your eye makeup. Dip a clean cotton ball in your foundation and then gently roll it over your eyeshadow. This will remove the eyeshadow only. Or, sweep a damp makeup sponge over the eyelid to tone down the color.

CREASE WEAR

Creamy eyeshadows are renowned for creasing after several hours' wear. To overcome this, use an oil-free foundation as a pre-makeup base on the eyelids. Some makeup artists advise setting cream eyeshadows with a dusting of translucent powder to help them stay put. Or, just smooth your fingertips over your eyelids every few hours.

PERFECT PORES

If your pores are large, you can camouflage them by applying foundation with a foundation brush. First, stroke the product in the direction of your nose. Then work in the opposite direction. This will effectively fill in your pores and give you the appearance of smoother skin.

BLUSH STROKES

To ensure that you never apply too much color, choose a shade that mimics your face after you've been exercising. But if you overdo your blush, either top with a translucent powder or simply swipe away a bit of the color with a tissue and a dab of moisturizer. Allow it to absorb before reapplying.

follow quick-fix solutions to rectify mistakes

UNEVEN LINES

If, after applying, you find your pencil or liquid eyeliner is not straight or the line is thicker in some spots than in others, use a cotton swab to smudge the line. To ease application, steady the hand using the eyeliner on a hard surface and look down into a mirror while you work.

LIFT OFF

Overly made-up brows will not create a very flattering finish. If you realize you have been too heavy-handed with your pencil while defining, make your brows look more natural by running a cotton swab over the top to lift off some of the color. Then wipe your index finger over them, brushing the hairs in the opposite direction of their natural growth, and finish by reshaping.

LIGHTEN UP

Dark lipsticks do not suit everyone. If you have applied your lip color and found it is too dark or does not go with your total makeup look, tone down the color by coating the lips with gloss and then blotting the color away using a tissue. Or, massage a small amount of beige or gold lipstick on to the lips as a top coat to lighten the color.

COLOR CORRECTORS

Color-corrective creams can be applied under foundation to alter your skin tone. If you're very ruddy, opt for a green color corrector. If you're sallow, lilac can brighten up your complexion. Use color correctors sparingly and blend so that they go undetected.

BEAUTY INTELLIGENCE

1

To create the illusion of greater lash length, plant a mascara wand at the base of your lashes and gently roll it horizontally as you glide it through the lashes.

Always use a light touch when applying mascara to your lower lashes, remembering that if you have small eyes this can easily make them look enclosed.

2

For the best results, opt for lip and cheek colors that are in the same color family as your eyeshadow to ensure that your overall look is not unbalanced.

3

If you have thin lips, stay away from dark lip colors and opt for glossy finishes. If you do go for a dark color, skip liner and top with a sheer or iridescent gloss.

4

A clever play on color can make the lips look soft and yet dramatic at the same time. Blend different shades of one color for an interesting finish.

5

If you don't have time to define your brows, apply a tiny amount of hairspray to your finger, and use it to keep unruly hairs in place.

6

Once you have applied your lipstick, seal in the color and simultaneously protect your lips by painting over them with a fine top coat of vitamin E oil.

7

Apply eye gel under your eyeshadow to act as a makeup base and condition the delicate skin around your eyes. Allow it to absorb before applying color.

8

If your favorite lip color does not have SPF, try layering on a lip balm with an SPF of 15 or higher first. Blend with your finger for an even finish.

9

To improve the staying power of your foundation, smooth on a primer first and allow it to absorb. Or, pat a translucent powder over your foundation and let it set.

10

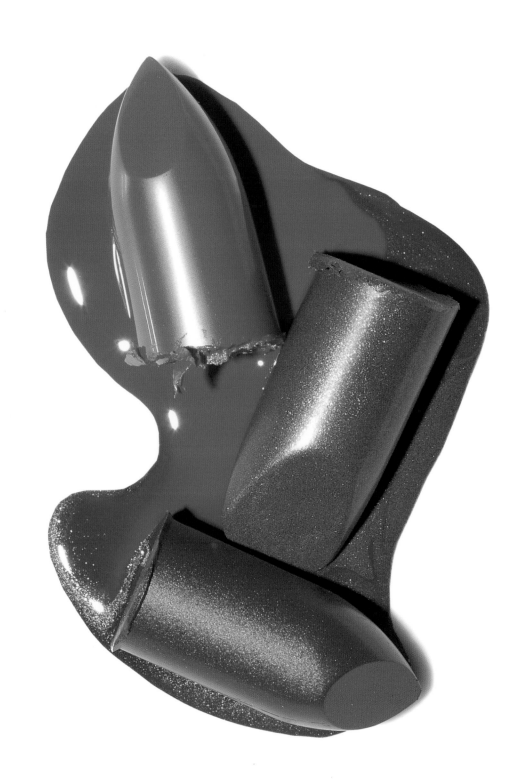

4

color choice

Color can say a lot about your personality and mood. For example, red may indicate that you are outgoing; pink can suggest femininity; green may reflect sincerity and balance; and violet can give the impression that you are artistic. Choose your hues to match your mood, but also look for shades that comp-lement your natural coloring.

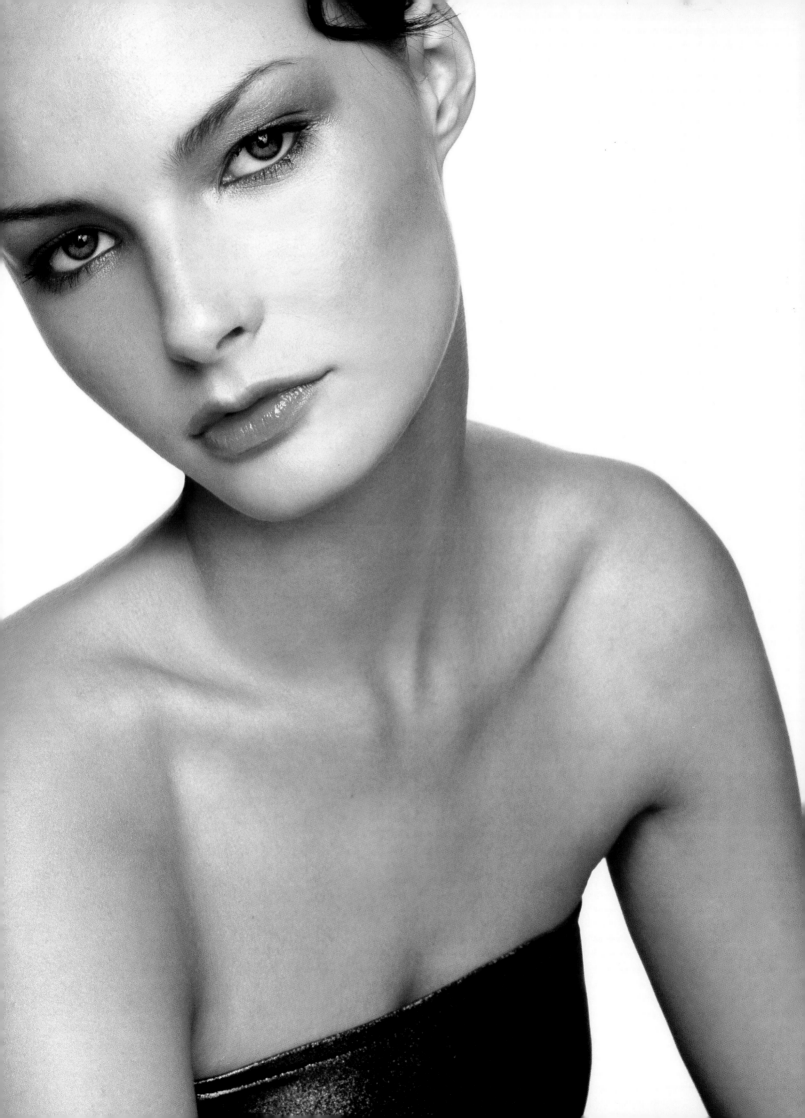

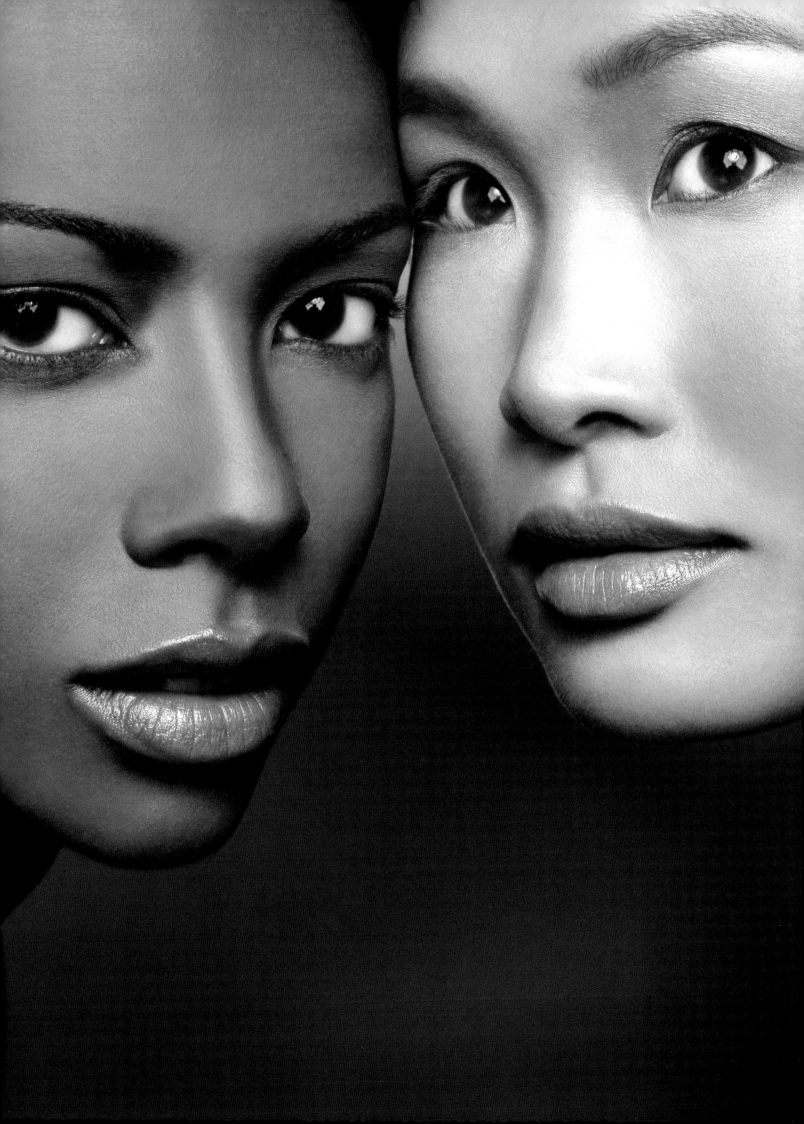

FAIR SKIN

Don't be tempted to use foundation in a shade darker than your natural skin tone to give more color. Instead, opt for makeup that has subtle yellow undertones to warm up your skin, and avoid anything too pink because it will end up looking ruddy. If you want to look lightly sun-kissed, sweep on blush that is peach or sheer bronze. If you're after a healthy, natural flush, try something in pale pink. For the eyes, navy blue, terracotta pink, silver, gray, and soft pastels like lilac and sky blue will suit you. On your lips, nude, rosy brown, beige pink and sheer red are especially pretty choices.

MEDIUM-TONED SKIN

This is the most common skin tone among Caucasian women and is best complemented by a foundation that has a yellow undertone. It is important not to go too light, as that will wash you out, or too dark, which will look unnatural. For your cheeks, try muted tawny and rose shades. Avoid anything with a strong orange base. On your eyes, go for beige, slate, moss, bronze and mushroom shadows—they're very flattering. On your mouth, try a berry-tinted gloss if your lips are naturally very pink. Or, for a more dramatic look, try plum, reddish brown, sheer chocolate and deep red lipsticks.

OLIVE SKIN

Your skin looks best with warmer tones of makeup. Pink- or orange-based foundations, especially, can look very mask-like. Your best bet is to find a yellow-based shade that is not too dark. For your cheeks, brownish rose and cocoa brown shades look good, but avoid bright red or orange. You may also want to play up your coloring with gold or bronze highlighters. For your eyes, choose reddish brown, deep purple, midnight blue and green. Avoid pearly whites and taupes, which may look ashy. For a beautiful mouth, try natural lip colors like rosy beige, deep red and sheer brown.

DARK SKIN

Generally, very dark to medium-dark skin needs a red/yellow-based foundation. Lighter-toned skin looks best in soft gold. Avoid makeup with titanium dioxide—it can make your skin look ashy. Using a highlighter around the hairline after applying foundation can keep this area from looking flat. For cheek definition, apricot, rose and bronze enhance lighter skin; deep plum, currant and dark rose suit medium to dark skin. On your eyes, try matte shades of brown and burgundy or shimmery shades of gold, bronze and silver. For the lips, red, burgundy, blackberry, peach, purple and caramel are all gorgeous.

ASIAN SKIN

You should use a yellow-based foundation and powder; anything with too much pink can make you look washed out. If you have a medium to deep skin tone, try tawny or rose blush, and avoid bright pinks and oranges, which will look garish. If your skin is light, try rose, sheer red or caramel. For your eyes, neutral shades like brown, black and gray are all great picks. On your lips, raisin, plum with brown undertones, red and mauve look best.

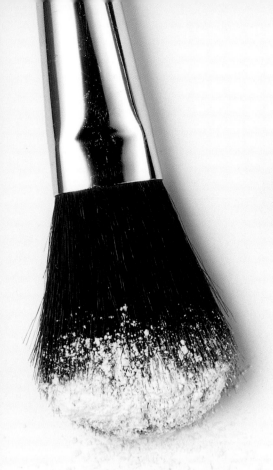

1

BLUE

Blue is no more or less wearable than any
other color. In fact, thanks to the wide range
of available shades—from dark cobalt to
sheer turquoise—it may even be among the
most universally flattering. Generally
speaking, mature women look best in
deeper tones, while younger skin can easily
pull off sheerer, more shimmery shades. But
if you just can't warm up to the thought of
blue eyeshadow at any age, try a navy
mascara or eye pencil instead.

2

PURPLE

Choose from the palest tone of lavender,
heather or violet to shade the eyes, and use
richer, stronger shades of blackberry and
deep plum to color the lips. If you're
wearing purple on the eyes, makeup artists
advise using just one color over the lid and
defining the lash line with the same shade in
a deeper tone. To balance the face, use
colors for the lips and cheeks that are of a
similar depth to the eyes, so the overall look
is not too heavy. Create an interesting
lipstick finish by applying a layer of gold
under deep plum.

3

PINK

Pink will suit most skin tones if you pick the
right shade. The color is very flattering to
younger skins and can be used as a wash
of color on the cheeks, lips and eyes. You
should avoid wearing pinks if your skin has
a tendency to look ruddy. And, on your
eyes, makeup artists advise sticking to
sheer pinks to illuminate your look.

six secrets for wearing color successfully

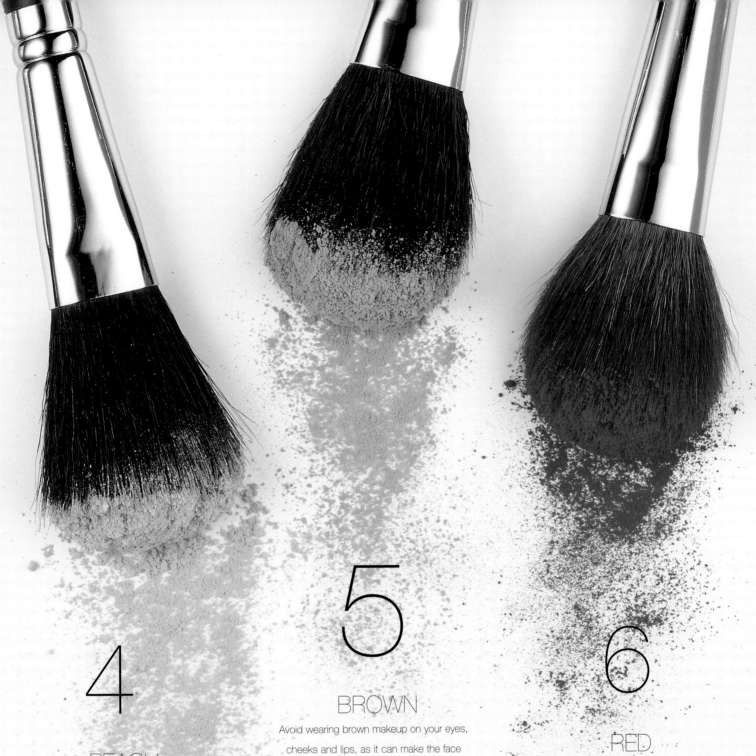

4

PEACH

Coral, apricot and peach are extremely flattering on the skin as long as they have a yellow undertone. They are a new way of creating a natural look, especially if you are stuck in a rut and always wear brown. Look for pale rather than orangey shades. Do not match lips, nails and cheeks by defining with the same color; look instead for different varieties of the same shade to create a more flattering effect. Avoid flat, opaque finishes and go for glossy, shimmering textures that impart luminosity to the skin.

5

BROWN

Avoid wearing brown makeup on your eyes, cheeks and lips, as it can make the face look dull. Spice things up by incorporating warm tones of terracotta, gold and copper into your palette, and go for a combination of different textures and finishes to give your features definition. If you have medium-toned skin, don't wear shades of brown that are too pale, as they can leave you looking washed out.

6

RED

Unless you're following a new fashion trend, wear red only on the lips, where it can make a strong beauty statement, especially if you have pale skin. When selecting a lipstick, avoid cool or bluish reds if you have red or golden-brown hair, as they can look dated. Blondes can wear any shade of red, but those with olive skin should opt for brown-based or wine and blackberry shades, while those with dark skin should choose mahogany. For a soft approach, use a sheer red lipstick to add a hint of color.

TEXTURE TWIST

Makeup is now available in every conceivable texture to give the skin a range of flattering finishes. The secret is to perfect your method of application: if you opt for total shine, you could end up looking a little greasy unless you are a professional; on the other hand, matte makeup can leave your face looking flat and lifeless. For the best results, aim for the middle ground and attempt a combination of matte and shimmering makeup on the face. Try teaming glistening skin with matte lips and shimmery eyes, or a matte complexion with metallic eyes and glossy lips.

SHINING TRUE
The new generation of shimmery makeup gives a soft finish that captures the light in a flattering way. You can choose from iridescent face and body powders, pearlized blushes, an array of metallic eyeshadows, lip tints and shimmery nail colors. Skin should glow without looking sparkly. There is a crucial difference between gleam and glitter. To give your skin a glistening finish, you can mix a shimmer cream with your foundation before smoothing it on. To achieve a natural look, apply shimmer to the areas of the face which normally catch the light, such as the tops of your cheekbones. If you have very oily skin, do not try to achieve a glistening finish or you could end up with a greasy look. Instead, use an oil-free foundation that dries to a matte finish, then slick on lip gloss or use an iridescent cream eyeshadow on the eyelid. To break up shimmer on the face, you can use a matte kohl pencil to add definition to frosted eyes or pair iridescent eyes and lips with a matte blush. For a subtle finish, experiment with shimmery eyeliners. These can give the eyes a flattering finish if they're in a light shade, like silver or soft blue. Just apply on the inner corners of the upper and lower lashes and blend out to fade gradually. When shopping for lipsticks, look for a shimmery finish that contains fewer reflective pigments. It will be much more flattering than any of its frosted counterparts, which have more pigments and yield a chalky effect.

MATTE MAKE-OVER
Matte makeup is the perfect way to offset high shine. Most makeup kits contain matte eyeshadow for shading and contouring the eyes. Matte pencils add definition to frosted eyes, while matte blush complements a shimmery highlighter. Matte lipsticks look great but some have a drying effect on the lips; also, as they wear off, they can leave an unsightly stain on the lips. One simple way of geting around these problems is to choose "semi-matte" formulations.

TEXTURE TRANSFORMATION
There are several simple steps you can follow to either transform matte products into shimmering finishes or turn high-shine products into matte formulations. One of the easiest ways to convert any matte product, whether it is lipstick or eyeshadow, into a glossy finish is to mix it with Vaseline or lip gloss. If you want to create a more subtle shimmer, simply sweep a wash of pearlized ivory highlighter over eyeshadow, blush or even lipstick. To tone down high-shine lipstick, press face powder onto your lips using a powder puff or blot your lips with a tissue to remove the glossy finish and leave just a stain of color.

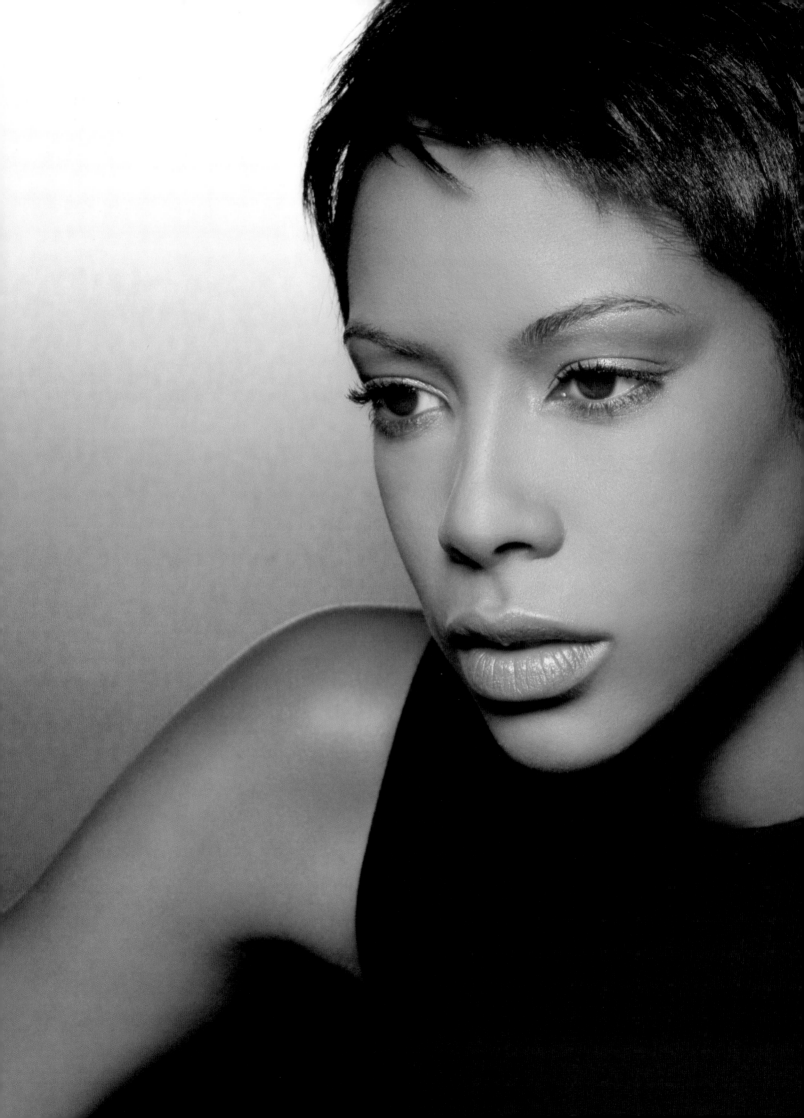

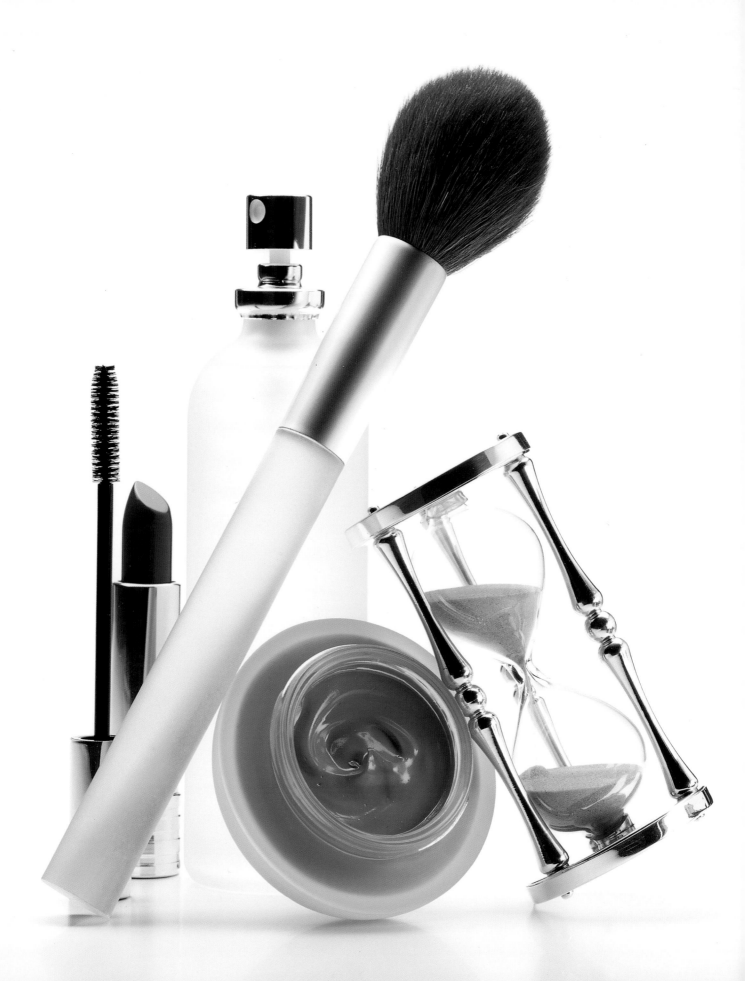

MATURE FACES

FOUNDATION As we age, our skin changes, becoming much drier and more prone to flushing. The tone is less vibrant, fine lines and wrinkles are more apparent, and the lips lose their fullness. Look for cosmetics that will flatter your skin's condition and color as it matures. Play up your strong features and use cosmetics to draw attention away from fine lines and wrinkles. Drier skins will benefit from oil-based foundations. Look for creamy formulations that will glide on smoothly, so that you avoid dragging the skin. Always wear moisturizer as an undercoat to plump up your skin, and look for a formula that contains a sunscreen to help prevent photoaging. Concealer is one of the mature woman's greatest allies. It can be used in order to tone down flushed skin, to disguise broken capillaries, to mask changes in pigmentation and to minimize deep shadows. Stick concealers are the easiest to apply. You should always opt for yellow-based concealers to complement any skin tone. Ruddy-looking complexions can be evened out with green color-correcting bases.

BLUSH Cheeks that are prone to flushing and covered in broken capillaries should be defined with soft browns and peaches, rather than pinks, to avoid accentuating the redness. Wearing blush will also help to draw attention away from crow's-feet around the eyes. Creamy formulations can give mature skin a flattering finish. Makeup artists suggest that you avoid using face powder later in life, as it can emphasize fine lines and wrinkles. If, however, you want to use powder, choose pressed rather than loose, as it is easier to control during application.

EYES Be very wary of using bright colors or tricky color combinations, as they can make the eyes appear small and deep-set. Look for warm browns, taupes, olives, lavender and chestnut red to shade the eyes. Avoid dark eye colors—certain shades of dark gray can make the eyelids look very heavy, especially if you are prone to tired or sallow-looking skin. Eyeshadow one shade darker than your foundation is a great option for day wear. If you feel that your eyes are more "droopy" than they used to be, do not coat the eyelid with color but just sweep color in the crease and line below your lower lashes to "lift" them. Bear in mind that matte finishes are more flattering than pearlized, frosted ones as you get older. Steer clear of bright white frosted highlighters and shimmering shadows, and look for powdery eyeshadows as opposed to cream or gel formulations, as they will stay where they are supposed to and not crease into fine lines and wrinkles. Define sparse brows by applying eye pencil in small, feathered strokes rather than one line, which will look severe. Coat the eyelashes with a lash-building mascara.

LIPS If you want to draw attention away from your eyes, use a strong lip color. But remember that very dark tones can look hard and make small lips appear smaller. If you do opt for a bright lip color, take steps before application to prevent it from feathering into fine lines around the mouth: coat the lips with a lip liner (it contains waxes and little oil, which makes it stay put longer than lipstick), blot with powder and then smooth on your lipstick. Then, blot with a tissue and reapply lipstick.

EVENING BEAUTY

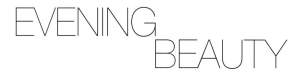

PREP WORK If you want your daytime look to take you right through to the early hours of the morning, follow these simple steps. Slip a cleansing wipe into your bag to use at the end of the day to freshen up your complexion and to remove what is left of your daytime makeup. Do not use it on your eyes or on the sensitive areas around the eyes; instead dab them with a damp cotton ball or with the tip of a moistened cotton swab to fix smudges.

MAKEUP BASE For a flawless evening base, apply a primer before foundation to smooth the skin and give your base something to adhere to so it lasts. Then, cover under-eye circles and blemishes with concealer.

P.M. GLAMOUR Beauty after dark is not about wearing lots of makeup in different colors. You should aim to look sophisticated in an understated way. Neutral daytime tones tend to disappear at night, so if you don't feel comfortable with the idea of drastically altering your makeup look, simply opt for the colors that you normally wear but choose slightly darker versions. This way, you will create a more dramatic effect but one that is not too far removed from your daytime look. Or, incorporate metallic—not glittery—finishes into your existing makeup palette. Blend gold with brown and copper, and silver with blue, pink and red.

NIGHT-TIME DRAMA For a modern look, make either the eyes or the lips the focal point of your face. If you try to accentuate both features, the results can look dated, harsh and artificial. If you choose to play up your eyes, use a wash of color on the lips. Or, paint on a strong shade of lipstick and simply run liner along your upper lashes, adding a couple of coats of mascara to finish.

SKIN LUMINOSITY Skin that is bared in revealing clothing should be given a radiant finish. Smooth on moisturizer and then dust with a shimmery powder or bronzing powder. For a golden glow, prime the skin with self-tanner a couple of days prior to your evening out. For the best results, smooth onto freshly exfoliated skin. The secret to a no-streak tan is to blend thoroughly. If you normally spend five minutes applying body moisturizer, take double the time with self-tanner—it will be well worth it. Don't forget the earlobes and the tops of the hands. If you end up with streaks, gently exfoliate the area or smooth on whitening toothpaste, leave on for five minutes and then remove.

FRAGRANT FINISH Perfume is a must for evening. Don't even think of dabbing it on behind the ears—the numerous oil glands located here can alter the balance of your perfume's ingredients. Instead, dab it on to the pulse points on the insides of your wrists, your cleavage or your nape.

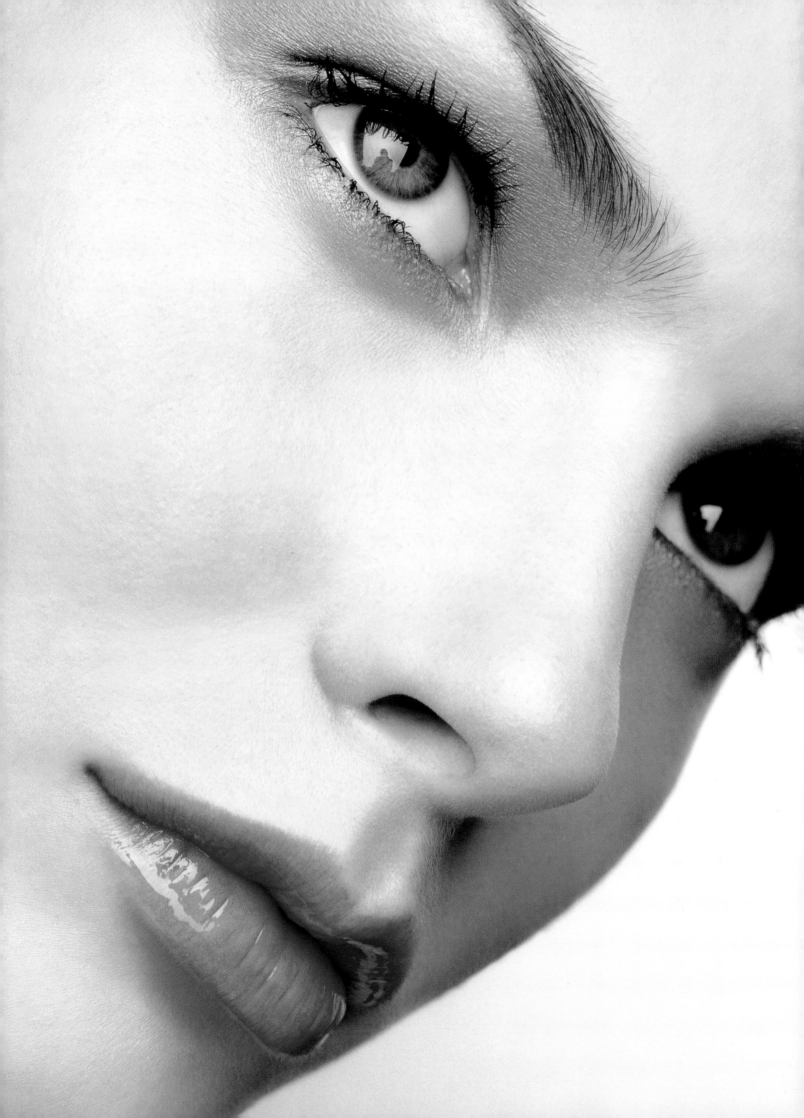

STAYINGPOWER

LASTING BLUSH

Dusting on powder blush takes a couple of seconds but it can disappear within hours of application. To improve its staying power, makeup artists recommend this foolproof tip: smooth on a cream blush and then dust with a powder formula in a similar shade. The powder blush will act as a setting agent over the creamy formula for lasting wear.

NAIL WORK

To make nail polish more durable, always apply a base coat before painting the nails with polish. This will create a finish on the nail surface, even when dry, which then acts as an adhesive base for the polish. Also, wearing a base coat helps to strengthen the nails and will prevent more brightly colored polishes from leaving stains.

LIP STAIN

Some makeup artists use a non-toxic, felt-tip water-based pen to stain the lips, creating a "bee-stung" that endures. You can get a similar effect from one of the many liquid lip and cheek stains now on the market. These products are typically applied with a tiny brush or sponge-tipped applicator. They dry very quickly and stay put; take them off with makeup remover.

SHADOW BOOST

You can always extend the staying power of your eyeshadow by smoothing an oil-free foundation onto the eyelids as a base before applying eye color. Oil-free formulations tend to glide on and not slide off, whereas their oil-based counterparts are not as long-lasting and therefore cannot provide a good adhesive base for eye makeup.

follow these steps to prolong the life of your makeup

LIPSTICK FIX

The new and improved long-wear lipsticks are the easiest way to get lip color that lasts. And, thankfully, most now come with a hydrating top coat so they don't feel as dry on your lips. A second option, though, is to just color in your lips with a flesh-toned lip liner, top with your regular lipstick, blot on a tissue, reapply the color, then blot a final time.

LASH POWER

You can improve the staying power of mascara by dusting your eyelashes with a little face powder before coating them with mascara. This will also make the lashes appear fuller and more voluptuous. If your mascara does not normally stay put, avoid wearing on the lower lashes and find a long-lasting formulation, as these are designed to be more durable.

BASE CONTROL

To improve the longevity of foundation, after applying a liquid formula, blot the face with a tissue. This will remove any excess surface oil that might interfere with the product's staying power. For maximum coverage, you can always add another thin layer of foundation and then finish off the look by setting this with a light dusting of face powder.

LASTING LINER

To make liquid or pencil eyeliner stay in place longer, after applying, trace the line with a fine brush dipped in powder eyeshadow or translucent face powder. The powder will set the eyeliner. Or, choose a waterproof formulation. These are more durable and contain special ingredients that are designed to withstand heat and humidity.

BEAUTY INTELLIGENCE

1 For a fresh, dewy complexion, avoid powder overload; apply it only to those areas prone to shine, like your nose, chin and forehead.

2 Make eyeliner application easier by lifting your eyelid at the eyebrow with one finger, so the skin is taut. Try to apply the liner in one smooth stroke.

3 If you want to use blush to give your cheeks a sculpted look, suck them in and softly contour the cheekbones, being careful not to create streaks of color.

4 In order to make your eyes look larger, makeup artists recommend that you leave a fine line between the edge of your eyelashes and your eyeliner.

5 As you get older, avoid metallic eyeshadows—glistening textures will only highlight fine lines and wrinkles. You will find that matte finishes are more flattering.

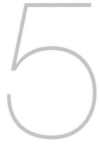

When choosing eyeshadow shades, it helps to consider the size of your eyes. If they're small, dark colors can make them appear smaller.

6

7

To give your pout definition, shade the outer corners of your lips with a pencil darker than your lipstick and dab lip gloss on the center of your lower lip.

If you want to downplay the size of your lips, skip lip liner, as this will accentuate their fullness, and go for a lip-toned lipstick.

8

If your complexion looks tired and lifeless, avoid foundation, which will only make things worse, and opt instead for concealer and tinted moisturizer.

9

Even if your skin isn't prone to clogged pores, look for foundations without mineral oil. This oil keeps skin from breathing and can cause breakouts.

10

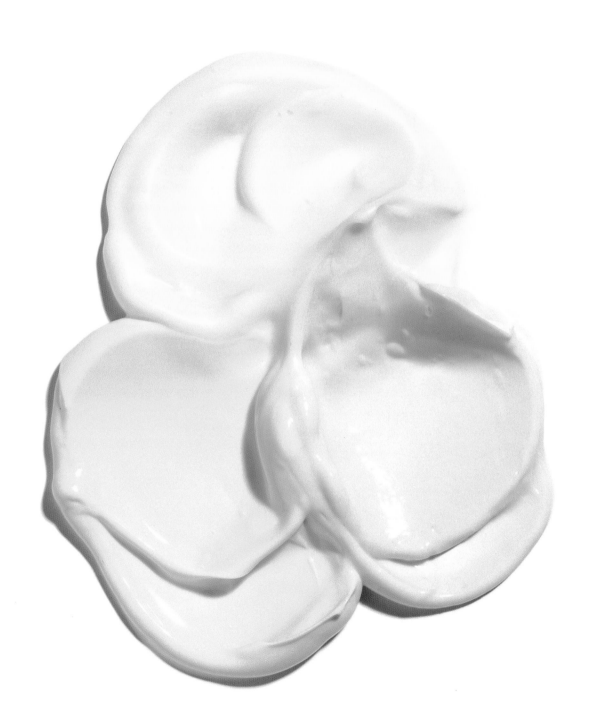

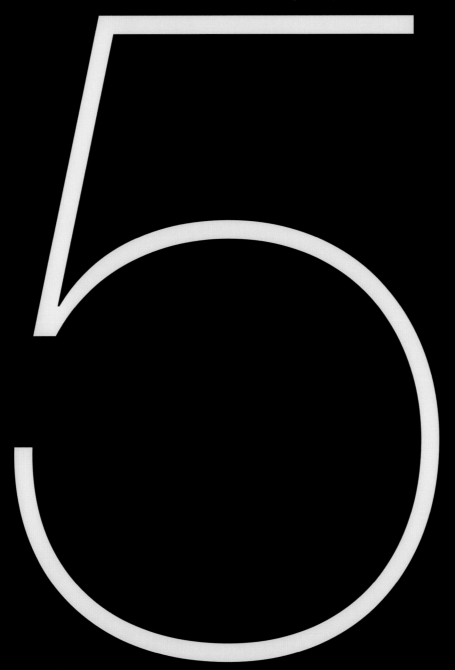

beauty upkeep

Good grooming might seem effortless, but there's a fine art to getting everything just right. It's not about sporting the most fashionable eye color or the latest lip gloss. The secret is to pay attention to the basics: your skin, nails and brows. If you follow the simple steps outlined in this chapter, you'll be well on your way to looking your best.

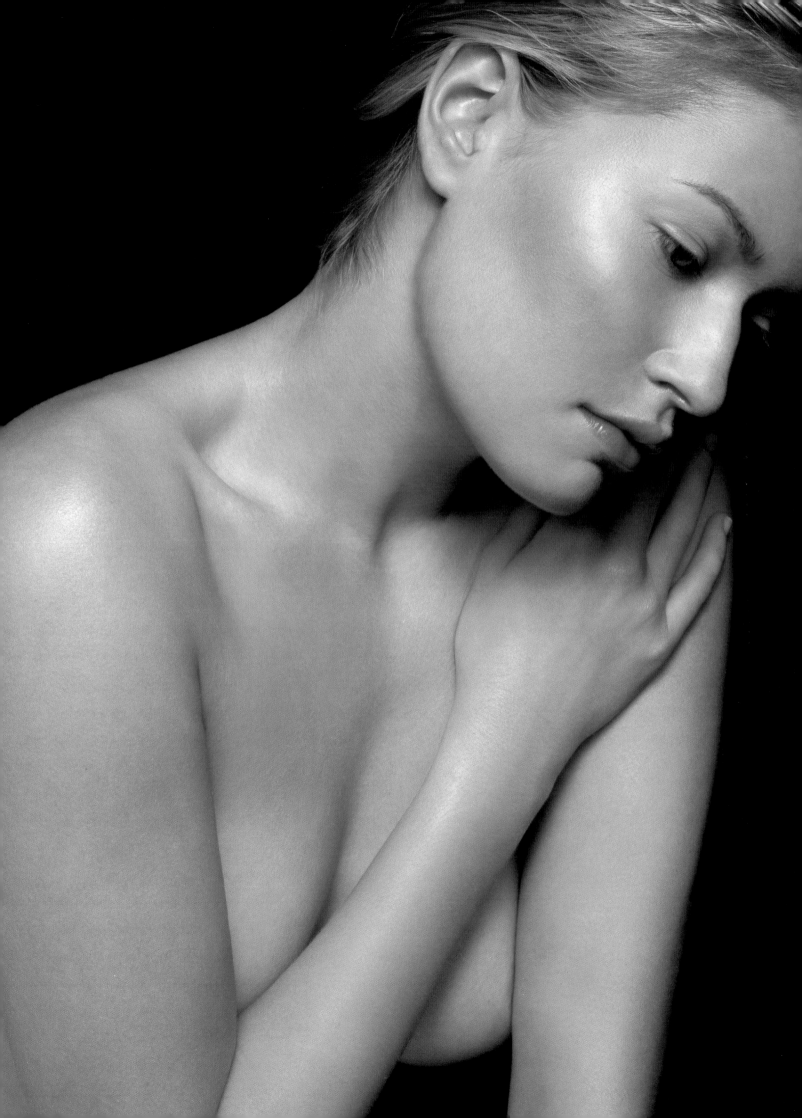

SKIN-CARE ESSENTIALS

EXFOLIATOR

should be used at least once a week to buff away dead skin and improve circulation. If you have delicate, sensitive skin, look for a formulation that contains special ingredients like enzymes or fruit acids that dissolve dead skin. Avoid those with granules, as they can be abrasive.

TONERS

such as floral waters are not a necessity but they can be used after cleansing or sprayed on as an instant pick-me-up. Avoid alcohol-based toners, which can strip the skin of essential moisture, causing dryness.

WASH-OFF CLEANSER

or a pH-balanced cleansing bar is ideal for use in the morning. Used with a facial cleansing brush or a washcloth, it can exfoliate and cleanse your face simultaneously.

EYE MAKEUP REMOVER

is essential for cleansing the delicate area around the eyes. Normal cleansers should not be used here, as they can contain fragrances and other ingredients that might irritate the eyes. Look for non-oily formulas and work gently from the outer corner of the eye inward, being careful not to drag the skin.

FACE MASKS

are a great way to enhance your skin's radiance. Those with oily skin will benefit from a once-a-week deep-cleansing face mask enriched with clay to help remove impurities and unclog pores. Those with dry skin should use a creamier, hydrating formula. If your skin is irritated and red, look for a fragrance-free mask labeled "calming."

CREAM CLEANSERS

or oil-based variants remove makeup and impurities and are ideal for use at night, as they are also slightly heavier than the rinse-off variety. Massage into the skin in small circular motions, and leave on for a few seconds. Remove with a washcloth or a damp cotton ball.

MOISTURIZER

used daily, is essential for all skin types. Look for a formula containing a sunscreen, as well as antioxidants to prevent premature aging, and sufficient hydration to suit your skin.

NIGHT CREAMS

are a good investment as the skin's recuperative and regenerative power is at its peak from 11 pm to 1 am. They generally contain special ingredients that will help this process.

EYE CREAM

can help protect delicate skin around the eyes. For day wear, choose a formula enriched with UV protectors and antioxidants. Gently pat into the skin under the eyes and along the orbital and brow bones. Don't apply it too close to your eyes or it might actually seep in and cause puffiness.

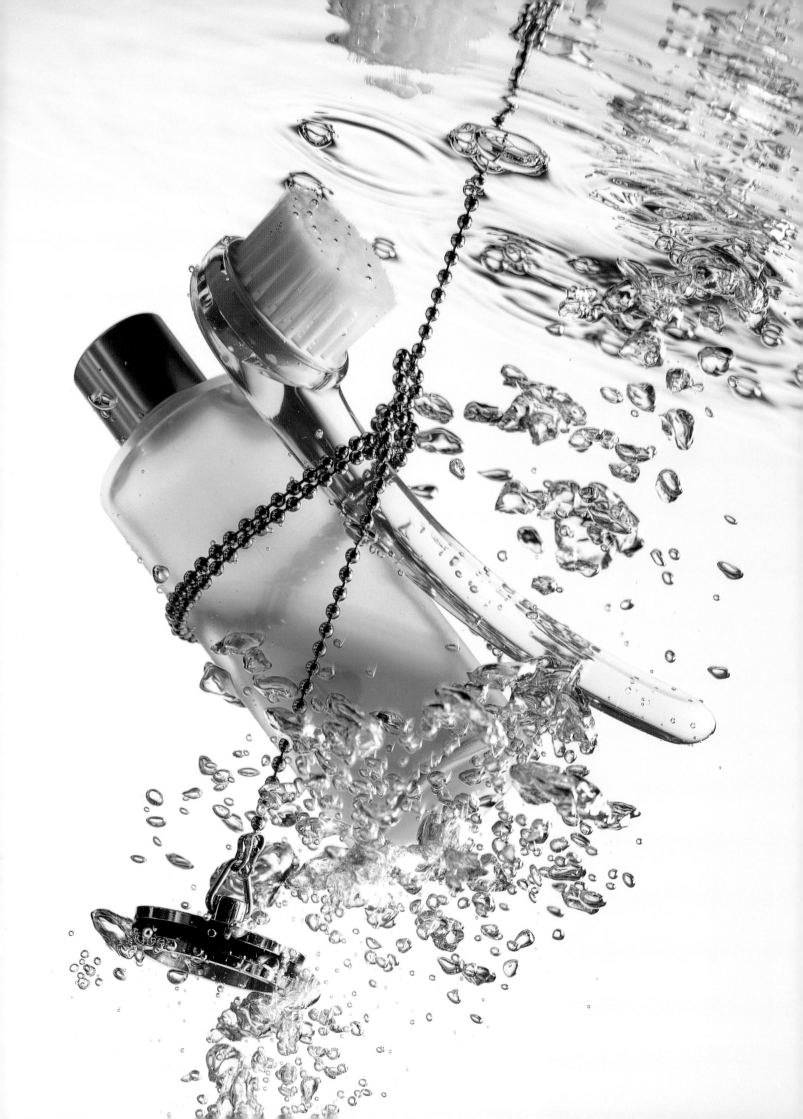

SKIN CARE

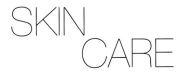

Whatever your particular skin type, there are three basic factors to bear in mind if you want a youthful-looking complexion. You will need to cleanse regularly, hydrate properly and provide your skin with protection from the elements. Your skin-care regimen doesn't necessarily have to be time-consuming or entail the use of lots of different products.

CLEANSING
Don't over-cleanse the skin. Skin is meant to act as a barrier, keeping irritants out and moisture in. When you over-cleanse, you strip away essential lipids and cellular matter that are responsible for retaining the skin's moisture. This can lead to heightened sensitivity, which in turn can result in mild redness, rashes and dermatitis. Over-cleansing can also cause dehydration and even adult acne. It may seem counter-intuitive, but by cleansing too frequently, or with harsh products, you can strip the skin of oil, which sends your oil glands into overdrive.

HYDRATING
Find a moisturizer that suits your skin type (more on that below), and don't be afraid to spot-apply it where necessary.

PROTECTING
The sun is the skin's deadliest enemy, responsible for about 90 percent of premature aging. Always protect your skin with a product containing an SPF of at least 15—remember, even on the most overcast days the sun's ultraviolet rays will penetrate the clouds. If you must have a bronzed look, incorporate a self-tanner into your beauty regimen.

OILY SKIN
Look for products, such as mattifiers, that control oil production. It's best to go for a gel-based cleanser, and an oil-free moisturizer as well. Don't skip moisturizer all together or you'll end up with dehydrated skin, which can look and feel uncomfortably taut. Plus, lack of hydration can actually exacerbate acne; when dry skin flakes trap debris in pores, you'll end up with blemishes.

DRY SKIN
Dry skin is either hereditary or occurs as a result of harsh weather, exposure to the sun or age. Invest in a rich moisturizer and use a creamy cleanser. Do not use alcohol-based toners. Exfoliate regularly, as a buildup of dead dry skin can prevent your moisturizer from being absorbed.

SENSITIVE SKIN
Your skin type usually feels tight and looks blotchy. It can flare up after trying new products, sun exposure or as a result of harsh weather. Avoid fragranced products or those with unnatural colorants, alcohol or chemical sunscreens. Choose creamy cleansers and shield your skin with products containing a physical sunblock like titanium dioxide. Avoid products with alpha hydroxy acids (AHAs). Networks of broken blood vessels can appear on your nose and cheeks. Take preventive steps by using sunscreen and a rich protective barrier cream. Avoid exposure to extreme weather conditions, spicy foods and hot water, all of which can exacerbate your condition.

COMBINATION SKIN
This type is usually oily in the T-zone and dry elsewhere. Most products for combination skin are formulated to work on surface dryness while controlling the underlying oiliness. Use a moisturizer that contains water and lipids, not oil; oil-free makeup; and gel cleansers. Avoid alcohol toners. Instead, go for those with AHAs to exfoliate and prevent clogged pores.

SKIN RADIANCE

PROFESSIONAL TOUCH If you can, treat yourself to regular facials every six weeks. Avoid having facials during your period, as the skin is more prone to sensitivity then. After a facial, try not to wear makeup for at least two hours to allow your skin to breathe.

BACTERIA ALERT Every time you open a jar of face cream or a bottle of lotion and dip your fingers in, you are introducing bacteria, which can affect the product's shelf life. Bottles with pump dispensers offer a simple way of getting around this problem.

SPOT ATTACK If you have blemish-prone skin, avoid alcohol, caffeine, spices and foods containing iodides, like shellfish, as they can sometimes stimulate oil production. Some skin-care experts recommend applying a 10 percent benzoyl peroxide spot treatment to the area, two or three times a day. If your blemish is large and cyst-like, apply a warm compress to it several times a day. Contrary to popular belief, toothpaste doesn't banish blemishes.

SOAP STRATEGY Some people swear that using soap and water is the secret to successful cleansing, but the experts tend not to recommend this approach. Conventional soaps often leave an alkaline residue on the skin, which is hard to rinse off and can interfere with the efficiency of moisturizers. Always use a pH-balanced facial cleansing bar suited to your skin type and wet the skin with warm water first. When rinsing your face, use only warm water, as water that is too hot can irritate the skin and have a drying effect.

BEAT BLACKHEADS Blackheads are caused by sebum blocking the hair follicles, not a buildup of dirt. Blackheads get their color when the sebum oxidizes upon exposure to air. If your skin is prone to blackheads and breakouts, regular deep-cleaning facials can help, as can using products with salicylic acid or benzoyl peroxide. For extreme cases, a prescription for a stronger medication may be advisable.

MASQUERADE To maintain skin radiance, incorporate a face mask into your weekly beauty regimen. If your skin is oily, a deep-cleansing clay or mud mask will help. Dry skin will benefit from moisturizing masks with ingredients like hyaluronic acid, vegetable proteins, amino acids and essential fatty acids. Soothe irritated skin with a mask containing anti-inflammatory ingredients, such as camomile and sea algae. To boost normal or dull skin, look for an exfoliating mask that will buff away dead skin cells.

CLEANLINESS Always wash your hands before you touch your face and avoid touching your skin unnecessarily. Clean the handset of your telephone regularly: aestheticians suggest using an antibacterial wipe to remove the germs and bacteria that accumulate there, as these could cause irritation on the skin under the jaw and lead to breakouts.

WEATHER CHECK During the winter, if your skin is exposed to harsh weather conditions or you have to spend prolonged periods outdoors, smooth on an oil-based moisturizer. Don't use water-based moisturizers, which can literally freeze on the skin, disrupting its natural balance.

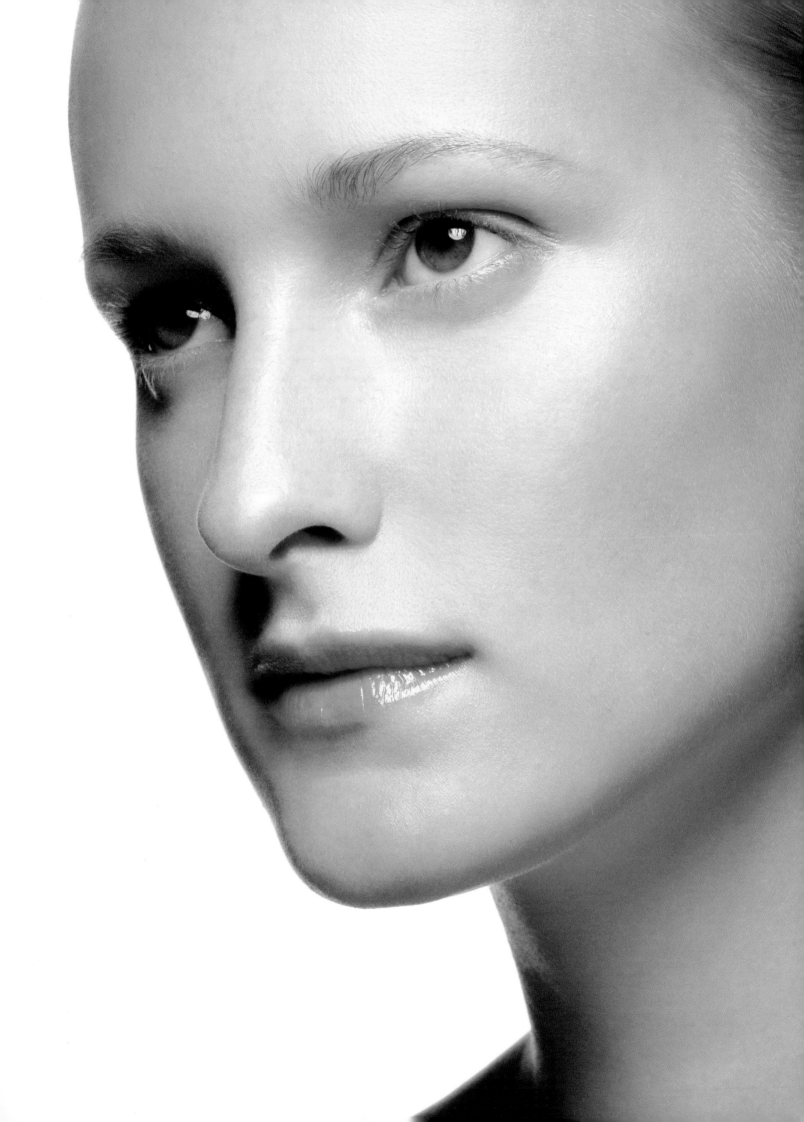

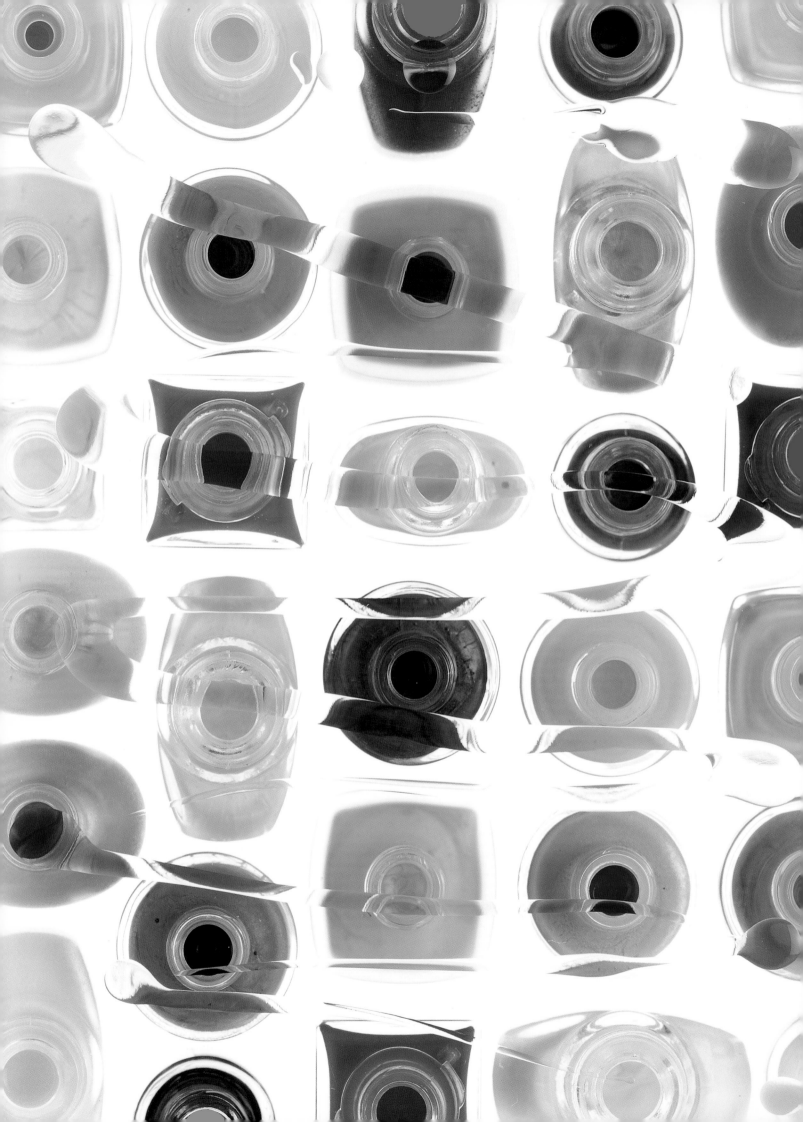

NAIL CARE

Nutrition plays an important part in the condition of your nails. Eat a well-balanced diet, including fresh fruits and vegetables, which provide vitamins and minerals, as well as poultry, meat, eggs and milk, which contain essential amino acids (the building blocks of hair and skin). While a low-fat diet is recommended by most doctors, an entirely fat-free diet can have detrimental effects on your skin and nails. White spots on the nails don't indicate a calcium deficiency; they are more likely to be caused by minor trauma to the nail. Gentle buffing can help.

SHAPE UP

Never file your nails after a bath or shower, as your nails are at their weakest then. Remember to work the file over the nails in one direction only, or you'll risk causing tiny tears that can lead to breaks. Short nails will stay neat-looking longer, whereas talons that extend way past the tips of the fingers are more susceptible to polish chips and breakage.

POLISHING TIPS

Before applying polish, always clean your nail beds with soapy water to get rid of any residue from nail treatments, as these can cause polish to bubble. Apply polish sparingly: the thinner each coat, the longer polish resists chipping. The first layer should be almost transparent. If polish has set on the skin surrounding the nails, swipe it off with a remover-soaked cotton swab. Never shake polish before application: this whips bubbles into the formula, which can lead to chipping when dry. Instead, simply turn the bottle upside down and gently roll it between the palms of your hands.

DISAPPEARING ACT

Before removing nail polish, massage a drop of oil or moisturizer into the cuticles. This will prevent them from drying out and stop the remover from setting the polish into your nails. There is still great debate about whether you should use acetone-free or acetone nail polish remover. Acetone polish remover is the most effective way to get rid of even the darkest colors, but it can cause nail dryness. To compensate, add a couple of drops of jojoba oil to the remover and shake well before using. If your nails become very dry, massage almond or jojoba oil into your nails twice a day.

COLOR CODE

Sheer colors are the most user-friendly and make imperfections less noticeable. When buying pale polish, take your skin tone into account: opt for pink or clear if you have a pinkish skin tone; beige, peach or clear suit darker skin tones. When choosing bright or bold colors, use the skin on the inside of your wrist as a guide to see if cool or warm tones suit you. If your skin has a bluish tinge, polishes with cool undertones will work; if it has a yellow tone go for warm colors. As you get older, avoid pale colors and natural shades since they can age the hands.

ONCE BITTEN

To put a stop to habitual nail-biting, have a professional manicure, then paint on one of those harmless but foul-tasting colorless formulas to discourage nibbling. Massage a drop of oil or cream into your cuticles and nails daily. If your nails start to look better, it will make you want to stop biting for good. Once you've broken the habit, use a hardener to get your nails into optimum condition, and treat yourself to manicures as often as you can. As your nails start to grow and become healthy-looking, paint the tips with a white matte or pearlized polish. This will make them look longer.

CUTICLE CARE

It's best not to trim your cuticles. Unless you do it properly, you'll be left with unsightly snags of skin around the nail, or worse, an infection. Instead, while you're in the bath or shower, gently scrub your nails with a soft-bristled nail brush. This will push back your cuticles, whisk away dead skin, rev up circulation and smooth the nail surface. Cuticle creams enriched with alpha hydroxy acids are good for keeping cuticles in shape. Manicurists recommend applying daily, preferably before bathing or showering, so that the heat can increase absorption of the cream.

HANDY TIPS

If you suffer from dry hands and brittle nails, avoid using highly perfumed lotions because the alcohol in them may leave your skin feeling even drier and irritated. When you are outdoors, use a hand cream enriched with sunscreen to prevent premature aging. Those with vitamin C can help prevent sun and age spots from developing. If these are already apparent on your hands, use a hand cream with hydroquinone on areas of discoloration. Never apply hand cream right after painting your nails, because this can dull the polish.

NAIL STRENGTH

If your nails are weak and prone to splitting and breaking, there are steps you can take to strengthen them. Try to use polish remover as little as possible; just once a week if you can. Protect your hands with rubber gloves when doing household chores, and make sure you eat a well-rounded diet, including plenty of protein (sorry, gelatin capsules won't help). Last, brush on a nail hardener daily, and don't forget to moisturize your cuticles every night. For maximum strength, keep your nails on the short side.

POLISH WORK

After you've removed your polish, if you are left with discolored nails, drop two denture-cleaning tablets into a quarter-full glass of water and use this solution to gently scrub your nails with a nail brush. Help prolong the shelf life of your nail enamel by wiping the rim of an open bottle with a little cuticle oil before replacing the top. This will stop the top from sticking and will also ensure that the bottle is closed properly. If the bottle is not airtight, the product will dry out and be unusable. Polish should always be stored in a cool place, as heat will expand the ingredients and can affect the product's consistency.

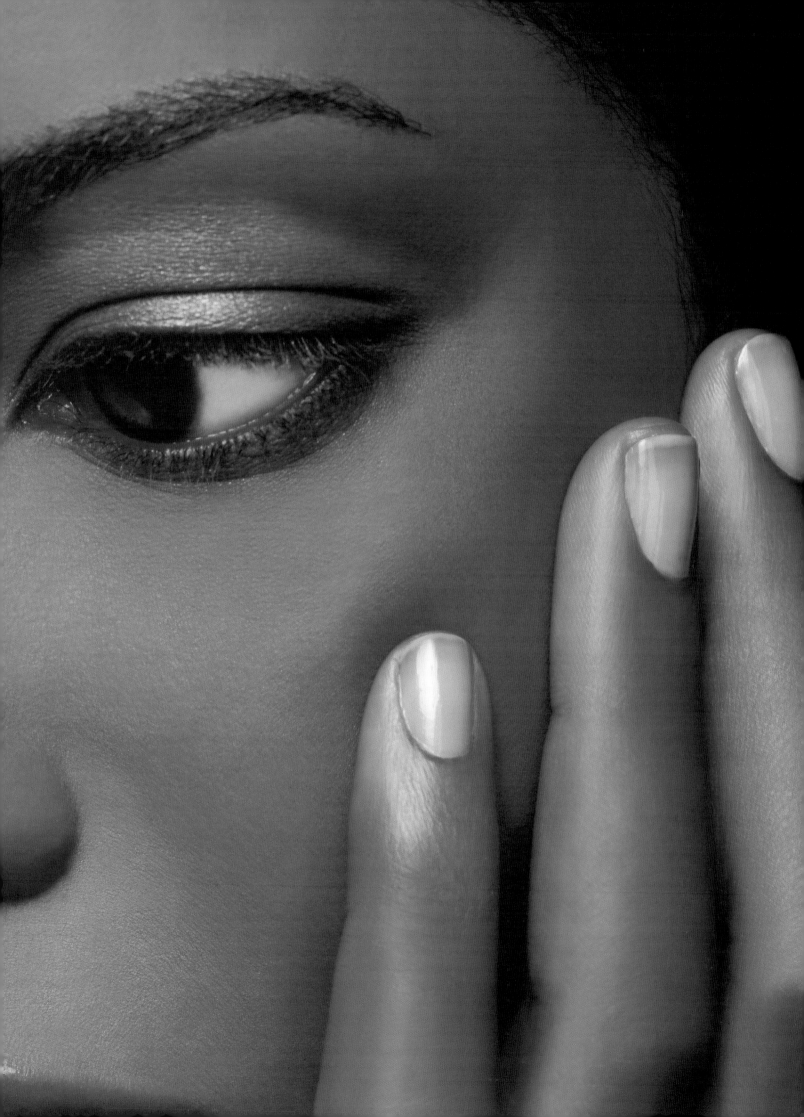

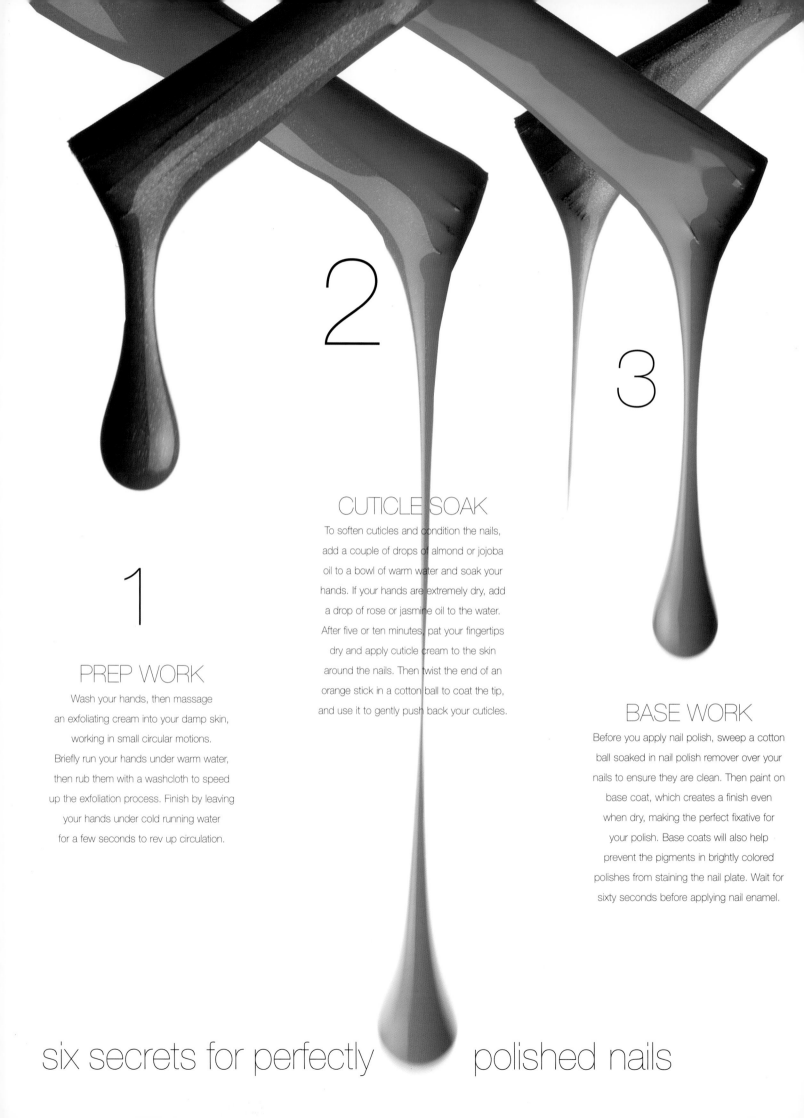

2

1

PREP WORK

Wash your hands, then massage
an exfoliating cream into your damp skin,
working in small circular motions.
Briefly run your hands under warm water,
then rub them with a washcloth to speed
up the exfoliation process. Finish by leaving
your hands under cold running water
for a few seconds to rev up circulation.

CUTICLE SOAK

To soften cuticles and condition the nails,
add a couple of drops of almond or jojoba
oil to a bowl of warm water and soak your
hands. If your hands are extremely dry, add
a drop of rose or jasmine oil to the water.
After five or ten minutes, pat your fingertips
dry and apply cuticle cream to the skin
around the nails. Then twist the end of an
orange stick in a cotton ball to coat the tip,
and use it to gently push back your cuticles.

3

BASE WORK

Before you apply nail polish, sweep a cotton
ball soaked in nail polish remover over your
nails to ensure they are clean. Then paint on
base coat, which creates a finish even
when dry, making the perfect fixative for
your polish. Base coats will also help
prevent the pigments in brightly colored
polishes from staining the nail plate. Wait for
sixty seconds before applying nail enamel.

six secrets for perfectly   polished nails

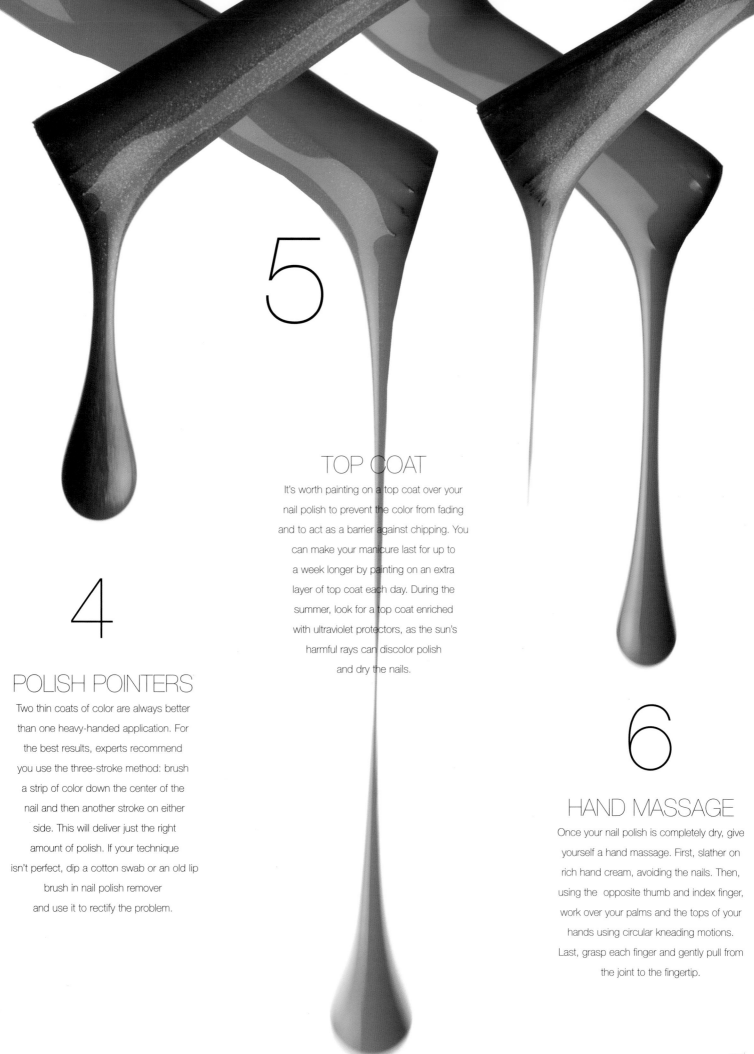

5

TOP COAT

It's worth painting on a top coat over your nail polish to prevent the color from fading and to act as a barrier against chipping. You can make your manicure last for up to a week longer by painting on an extra layer of top coat each day. During the summer, look for a top coat enriched with ultraviolet protectors, as the sun's harmful rays can discolor polish and dry the nails.

4

POLISH POINTERS

Two thin coats of color are always better than one heavy-handed application. For the best results, experts recommend you use the three-stroke method: brush a strip of color down the center of the nail and then another stroke on either side. This will deliver just the right amount of polish. If your technique isn't perfect, dip a cotton swab or an old lip brush in nail polish remover and use it to rectify the problem.

6

HAND MASSAGE

Once your nail polish is completely dry, give yourself a hand massage. First, slather on rich hand cream, avoiding the nails. Then, using the opposite thumb and index finger, work over your palms and the tops of your hands using circular kneading motions. Last, grasp each finger and gently pull from the joint to the fingertip.

EYE WORK
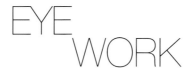

EYEBROWS Incorrectly plucked brows will throw your face off balance. If you haven't plucked them before, leave it to the experts for the first time. You can then master tweezing as your brows regrow, using the initial shape as your guideline.

THE PERFECT ARCH Tweezed brows should always resemble their natural shape. If you have small features, keep your brows quite fine and tapered; if you have small, deep-set eyes, a well-shaped arch will make them appear bigger. To achieve the perfect arch, hold a pencil vertically alongside your nose to just above your brow bone: this is where the brows should start. Twist the pencil diagonally from the base of your nose to the outer corner of your eye: this is where your eyebrow should end. Then hold the pencil vertically to the outer corner of the iris: this is where the peak of the arch should be. If you find it hard to shape your brows, draw in a guideline using an eye pencil before you start. You can wipe it off with cleanser.

TWEEZING Pluck hairs individually, clasping at the root and removing in the same direction as hair growth. If you pluck too many hairs from the outer corners, this can make the eyes seem close-set; if you over-tweeze at the inner corners of the eyes, they will seem too far apart. Only remove stray hairs from beneath the brow bone and between the eyes. Plucking hairs above the brows can disturb the natural line and make the eyes appear smaller. Be careful not to overpluck the brows as this can eventually diminish regrowth.

WAXING If you have extremely bushy brows or numerous hairs between the brows, you can have them waxed. It is a quick process, but should be done only by the experts and is more painful and expensive than tweezing. Hairs will grow back in about four to six weeks.

EYELASHES Apart from protecting your eyes, eyelashes can really accentuate your look when they are curled and defined properly. With age, eyelashes tend to lose color and become more sparse, which makes mascara a must.

CURLING Curling your eyelashes instantly opens up the eyes and adds definition to the face. Using a metal lash curler, clamp lashes near the roots, hold for several seconds and then release. Never curl mascara-laden lashes: as the mascara dries, lashes can stick to the curler and be torn from the roots.

FAKING IT Individual false lashes or strips cut to size can add definition. Run a small amount of clear lash glue along their edges, then, with a fingertip or tweezers, plant them by the roots of your natural lashes. To ease into place, use tweezers or an orange stick. If the glue shows, cover with mascara or liquid eyeliner. Coat false and natural lashes with mascara to bind them together. Always remove false lashes before going to bed.

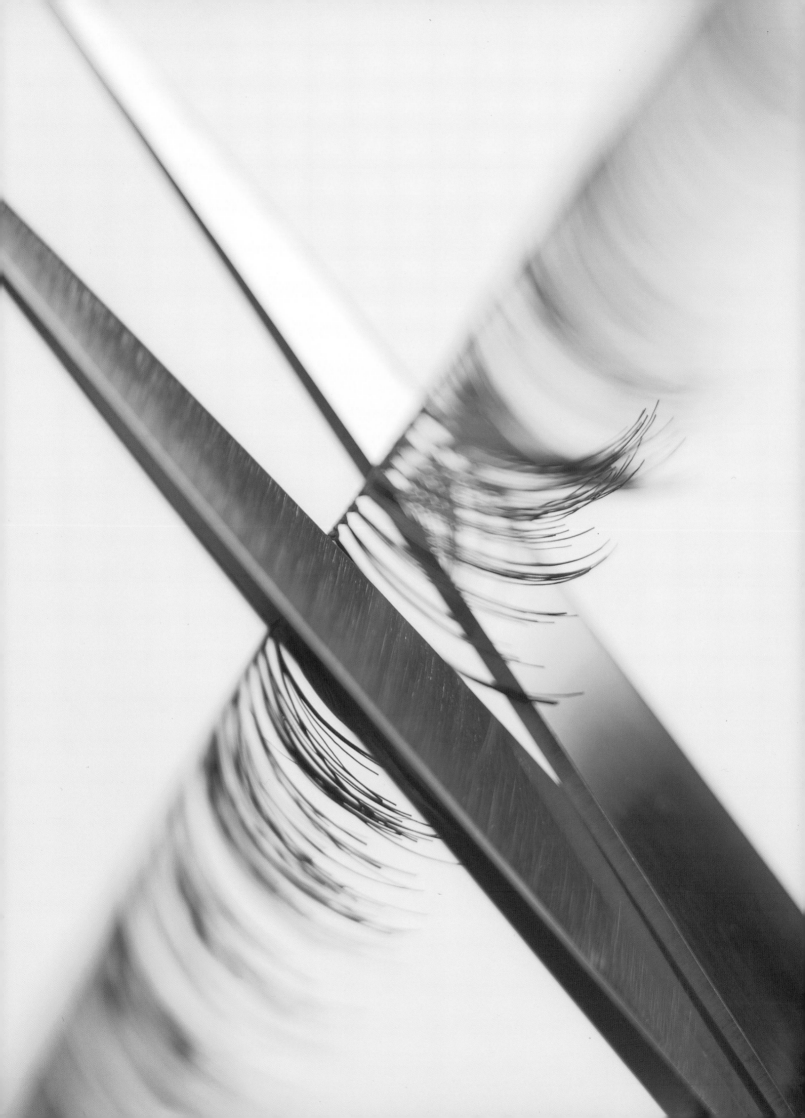

GOODGROOMING

FRESH-FACED If you want to look like you're not wearing foundation, but still need to conceal imperfections, try mixing a small amount of foundation with your moisturizer. Apply liberally to the face and neck, making sure that the product does not accumulate in your brows.

EYE RELIEF Dark undereye circles can be hereditary, or they can be caused by medication, stress or poor circulation. To counteract, pat on stick concealer a shade lighter than your skin tone. Puffy eyes can be caused by a bad diet, allergies and fluid retention. To shrink swelling, try a cold compress or elevating your head at night with an extra pillow.

SPOT FIX If you can't resist picking at your face, at least do it the "right" way: With clean fingers, gently pull the skin on either side of the blemish away from it (do not squeeze). If nothing comes out, leave the spot alone. Then top it with a spot treatment. To camouflage a blemish, paint concealer onto it with a fine-tipped makeup brush. Blend, then set with powder.

LASH BOOST If you're tired but want to look wide awake, add a couple of individual false lashes to the top outer corners of your eyelashes. Dip the end of each lash in clear lash glue, then plant the false lashes at the roots of your natural lashes. Once in place, hold until the glue sets. If the false lashes look like they are too long, trim to size before applying.

take short cuts to make yourself look good

LIP PRIMING
If you want a fresh-faced look with barely any makeup, keep your lips in good condition. For an exfoliating treat, smooth on Vaseline and then very gently run a toothbrush over the lips. Or, while you're using an exfoliator on your face, work the product over your lips, too.

FLATTERING FINISH
If your hands are not looking their best, this can affect your confidence and self-esteem. If you have sun and age spots or uneven skin tone on your hands, mix a long-lasting foundation with hand cream and massage this into the skin. Afterwards, wipe the palms of your hands with a tissue to remove any of the product that has not been absorbed.

TRESS WORK
If your hair looks greasy but you don't have enough time to wash it, work with your hair's natural oils and simply add some wax or hair gel to slick the hair back, or sweep it up into a topknot. Or, invest in a can of sprinkle-on dry shampoo to mask the greasiness. If you're not so time-pressed, wash your hair with a two-in-one shampoo and conditioner.

BROW DEFINITION
If you're not wearing makeup but want to look good, groom your brows. Brush them up and then comb into place to remove stray hairs. If you have fair hair, give brows definition to enhance your face. Dust on brow powder in a shade that matches your hair with a blunt-tipped brush or apply a pencil in small strokes and blend with your fingertips.

BEAUTY INTELLIGENCE

If you have sensitive skin, do not use any eye creams containing alpha hydroxy acids (AHAs) as they can cause irritation to the delicate area around the eyes.

If you have painted nails, avoid hand creams containing AHAs, which discolor polish. Instead, use a moisturizing face mask to hydrate the hands once a week.

Avoid permanently tattooing in brow color, which tends to look unnatural and can be a painful process. Instead, use a pencil to shape and define eyebrows.

Aim to tweeze your eyebrows after you've taken a bath or shower, since this is when the skin will be soft and your brows will be easiest to extract.

If you find that your eyebrow hairs have become too long, trim them with a pair of nail scissors before you pluck.

If you have had your hair lightened and want your brows to match, you can carefully bleach them at home, but it's best to leave this to the experts.

Don't throw out old mascara wands. They can be cleaned with soap and warm water and then used to tame your brows.

Every month, stop wearing nail polish for at least two days, to allow air to get to the nail plate. Then, give nails a high-shine finish using a nail buffer.

You should never use other people's mascara as this is one of the most common ways of contracting conjunctivitis and spreading other eye infections.

Instead of mascara, makeup artists often use tinted brow-grooming gel to define the lashes, as this adds thickness and color but looks more natural.

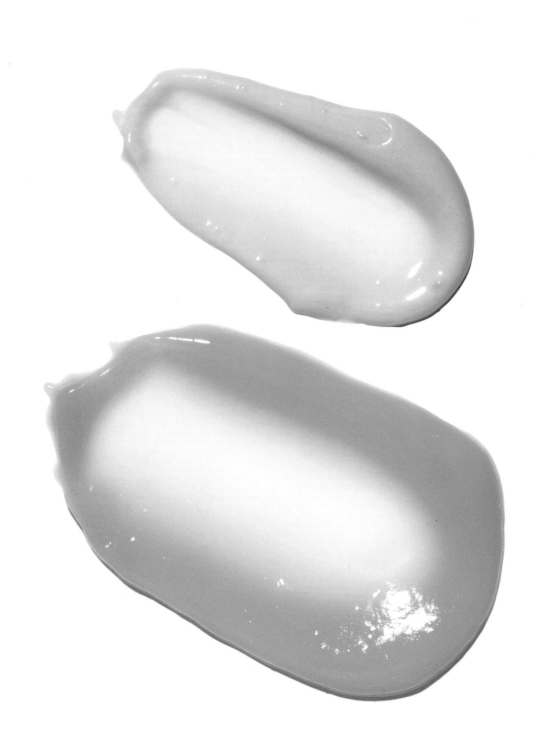

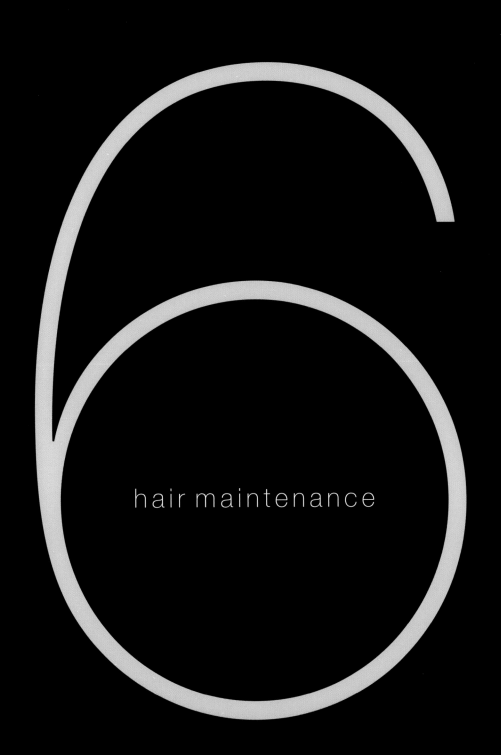

hair maintenance

Everyone can have great hair, even those of us not genetically blessed with thick, lustrous tresses. The secret to achieving healthy, gorgeous hair lies in combining the right maintenance regimen with the appropriate products—plus some professional styling advice. Then, keeping your hair in great condition should be quick and easy.

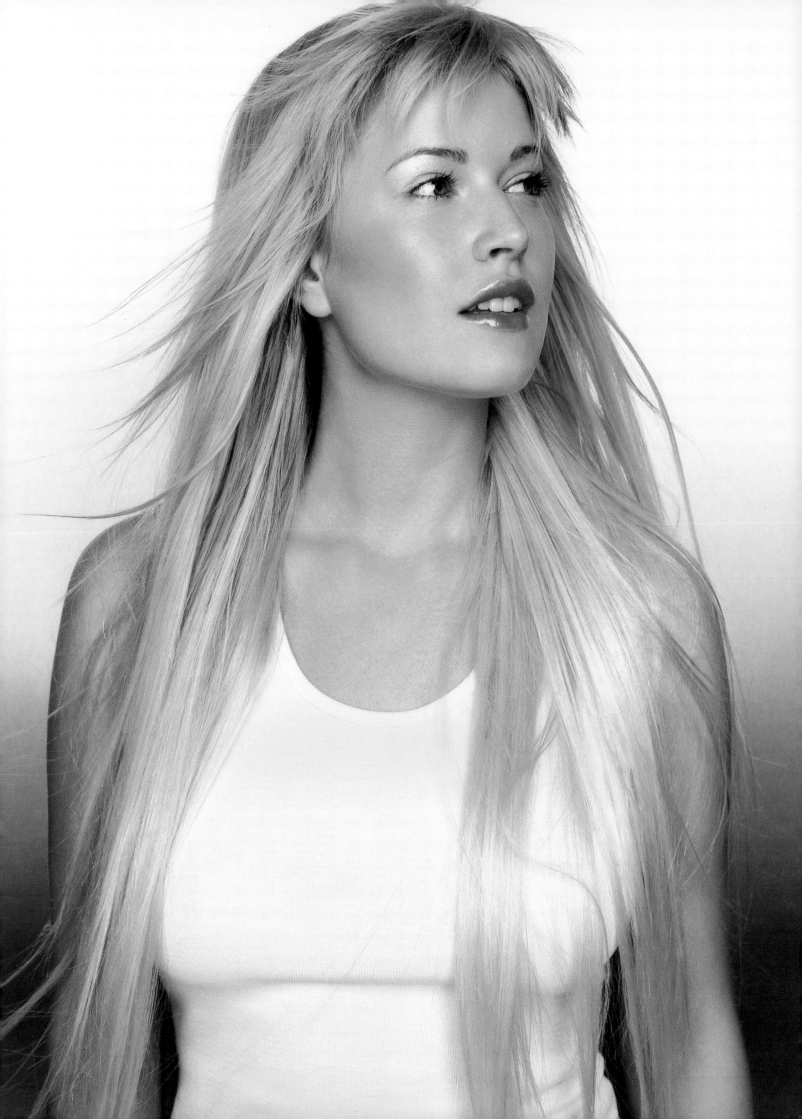

HAIR-CARE
ESSENTIALS

LEAVE-IN CONDITIONERS

are a no-rinse option for conditioning the hair and are ideal if you are pushed for time. They won't weigh down fine hair and help tame flyaway, frizzy hair. If the ends of your hair are extremely dry, you can smooth on a small amount of leave-in conditioner as a post-styling fix. This will help hydrate and protect the ends while improving their appearance.

SHAMPOOS

are surfactant-based creams or gels that emulsify dirt and oil in the hair, allowing them to be washed away by water. Most formulas use sodium or ammonium lauryl sulfate as their principal surfactant, then add ingredients to increase the shampoo's lathering power, treat the scalp, moisturize dry hair, etc. Look for a formula made especially for your hair type.

CONDITIONERS

should be used after shampooing. Typically designed to work within thirty to sixty seconds, conditioners coat and flatten the cuticles surrounding the hair shaft, creating an even surface to reflect light and give you glossier hair. This coating action also helps prevent snarls and makes combing easier.

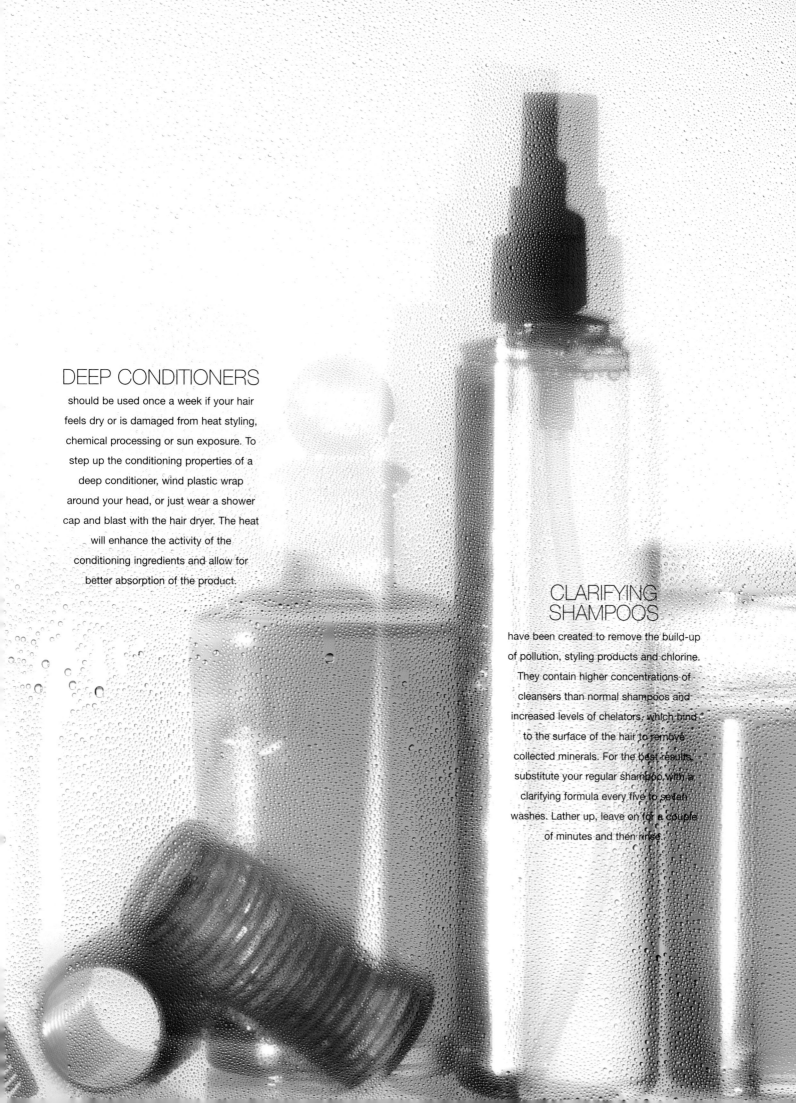

DEEP CONDITIONERS

should be used once a week if your hair
feels dry or is damaged from heat styling,
chemical processing or sun exposure. To
step up the conditioning properties of a
deep conditioner, wind plastic wrap
around your head, or just wear a shower
cap and blast with the hair dryer. The heat
will enhance the activity of the
conditioning ingredients and allow for
better absorption of the product.

CLARIFYING SHAMPOOS

have been created to remove the build-up
of pollution, styling products and chlorine.
They contain higher concentrations of
cleansers than normal shampoos and
increased levels of chelators, which bind
to the surface of the hair to remove
collected minerals. For the best results
substitute your regular shampoo with a
clarifying formula every five to seven
washes. Lather up, leave on for a couple
of minutes and then rinse.

HAIR TYPES

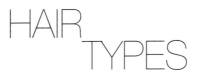

NORMAL If you are lucky enough to have been born with normal hair, look after it. Wash and condition it every day. Just because your hair is normal, this doesn't mean it's more resilient. Take measures to maintain its overall condition by using products that will protect it from heat styling and shield it from ultraviolet light. Get trims regularly to help prevent split ends.

DRY If your hair is dry, it is not receiving sufficient oil from the scalp. This can be the result of exposure to the sun, stress, dietary imbalances, chemical processing (such as coloring, relaxing and perming) or a hereditary condition. Try using moisturizing shampoos and conditioners to hydrate your hair. Give your scalp a pre-cleansing treat by massaging it with almond or jojoba oil (which is similar to the hair's natural oil). Leave the oil on for about ten minutes before shampooing. Brush your hair regularly to stimulate the scalp and to distribute the existing oils from roots to end.

GREASY Greasy hair is caused by overactive sebaceous glands that produce too much oil, known as sebum. Stress, poor diet, hormonal imbalances and harsh hair-care products can trigger the glands to go into overdrive. To remedy this, wash your hair daily with a mild shampoo, making sure that you cleanse the scalp effectively, and use a lightweight conditioner. Once a week, try rubbing jojoba oil (which is similar to the hair's natural oil) into the scalp and leave it on overnight. Adding oil like this will trick the hair into believing that it is producing the oil itself and so will help regulate the natural sebum production.

CHEMICALLY TREATED Relaxing, perming or coloring changes the hair's porosity, making it more susceptible to damage. You should always use shampoos and conditioners that are specially formulated for chemically treated hair—they are designed to maintain either the color or the curl of the hair. Use protein-enriched deep conditioners to help strengthen and repair the hair; these work by bonding to the hair shaft where the damage has occurred during chemical processing. Color-treated hair fades in the sun, so you should really wear a hat, or at least use products that contain sun protectors when you're outside in the rays.

COMBINATION It is very common to have active sebaceous glands which make the scalp and the roots of the hair greasy while the ends are dry, frizzy and prone to breakage. To deal with this problem, you don't need to spend a lot on a wide range of shampoos and conditioners. Instead, massage a mild shampoo into the roots, where grease accumulates and attracts dirt, and then use a wide-toothed comb to run it through the rest of the hair. Finish by working conditioner into the ends of the hair (avoiding the roots and scalp). Never have the water too hot, as this will stimulate the oil-producing glands.

COARSE HAIR Coarse, dry hair, common among African-Americans, is susceptible to damage and breakage, and, as a result, can be hard to handle. You should use intensive pre-shampoo treatments to help hydrate the scalp and the hair, massage the scalp regularly to encourage oil production, shampoo as often as necessary and deep condition once a week. If you feel you want to tame your hair, try relaxing. This is a chemical process that has the reverse effect as perming. Chemical relaxers are made in different strengths to suit different hair textures and styles.

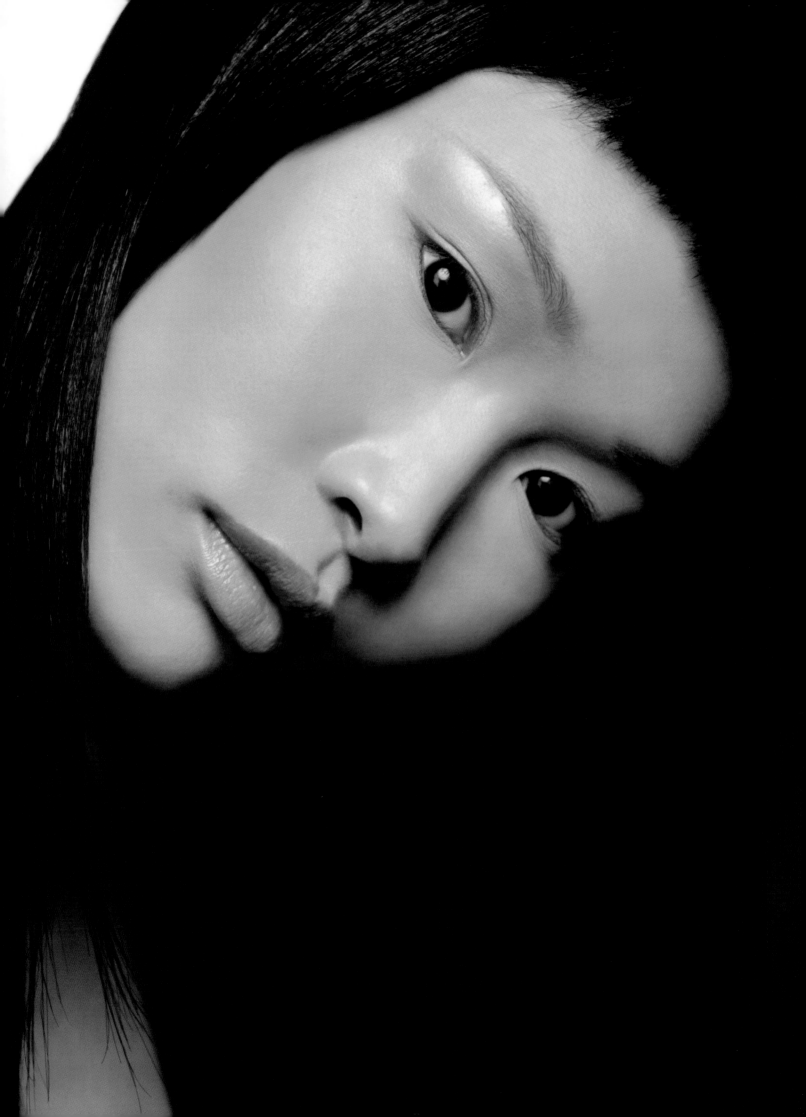

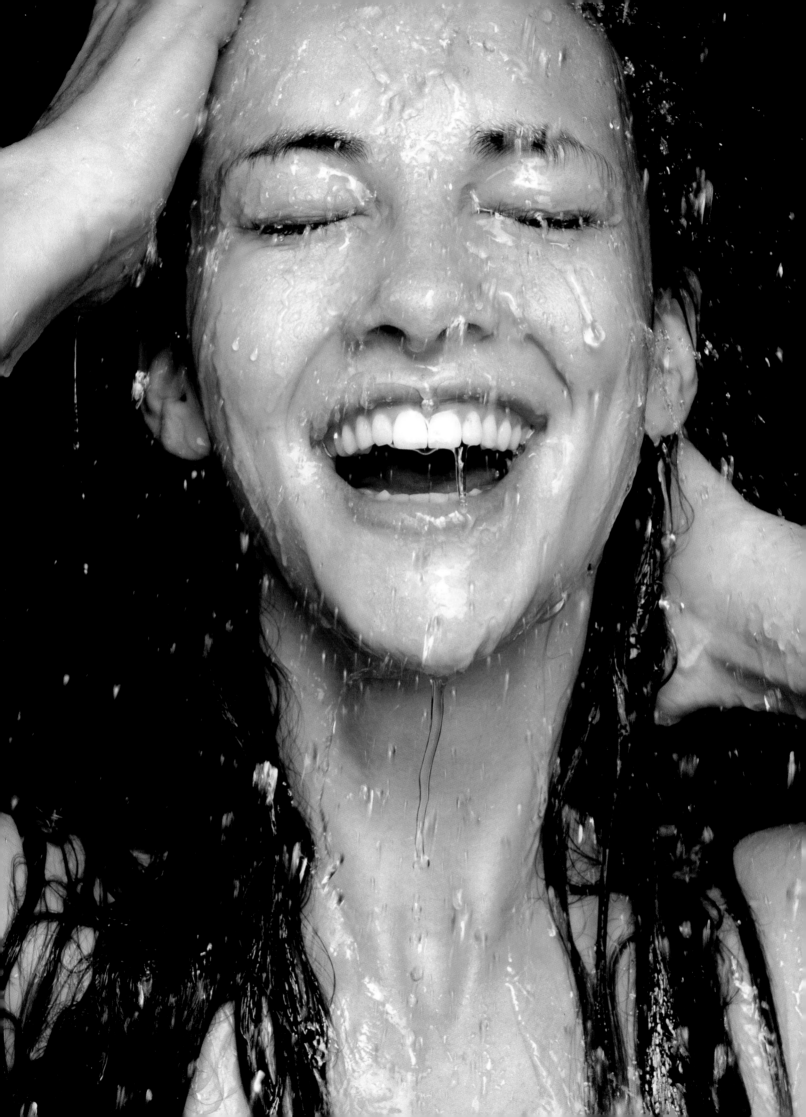

HAIR UPKEEP

CLEANSING Either look for a shampoo that is suited to your hair type or invest in a very mild (daily) formulation. If your shampoo doesn't lather into loads of suds and bubbles, this is not an indication that it will not cleanse the hair thoroughly. Never use too much shampoo, as over-washing will remove the hair's natural oils. If you wash your hair daily, one shampoo will suffice; if you insist on washing it twice, use only a small amount of shampoo. Keep the water tepid when you are washing your hair, as hot water can agitate the scalp and step up the activity of the oil-producing glands, making hair greasy. Before applying conditioner, blot excess moisture from the hair with a towel or squeeze with the hands.

CONDITIONING Conditioners play a vital role in maintaining the shine and general appearance of the hair. If you skip them, it can result in your cuticles not lying flat and your hair looking dull and lifeless. It will also be more susceptible to damage. Leave-in conditioners are ideal for people with short hair or those who don't want to spend too long on their hair-care regimens. You only need to apply conditioner from the mid-shaft to the ends of your hair, as the scalp's oil-producing glands usually supply the roots with sufficient moisture. After applying, run a wide-toothed comb gently through the hair, rinse thoroughly and finish with a blast of cold water. This ensures

that the cuticles will lie flat and provides a stimulating boost for the scalp. Do not towel-dry the hair vigorously but simply blot off any excess water; otherwise you will damage the hair and dishevel the cuticles. Never brush the hair when it is wet; always use a wide-toothed comb instead.

DEEP CONDITIONING If your hair is very coarse or dry and damaged from chemical processing, excessive heat styling or sun exposure, incorporate a deep-conditioner into your beauty regimen until your locks are restored to their former health. You will have to use your own judgment when deciding how often to go for this type of treatment, keeping in mind that one of the most common causes of lifeless-looking hair is over-conditioning. Protein conditioners rebuild the hair, as they are absorbed into the cuticle, strengthening the hair shaft, while moisturizing packs help hydrate and improve manageability. For the best results, use on freshly washed hair that has been blotted with a towel to remove excess water. To step up the conditioning properties of a hair treatment, slather it on before going into a sauna or steam room. If you're heading for the beach, it's a good idea to smooth on a deep conditioner, leaving the sun to activate the ingredients. This will protect your hair and also improve its overall condition.

FLAKY SCALP

Often confused with dandruff, flaky scalp occurs when surface skin cells slough off at an accelerated pace. This can result from poor circulation, not brushing the hair sufficiently, using harsh products or not rinsing shampoo off properly. To treat, use a mild or moisturizing shampoo, working into the scalp thoroughly. Also, avoid medicated shampoos, which tend to work only temporarily anyway and may contain ingredients that irritate the scalp.

DANDRUFF

Dandruff is believed to be the result of an overabundance of yeast called *pityrosporum ovale* on the scalp. (This yeast is found on healthy scalps too, just in smaller quantities.) The excess growth irritates the scalp's oil glands, causing them to shed skin cells at a faster rate, and leaving you with itchy flakes. To treat, look for a shampoo containing one of these FDA-approved ingredients: salicylic acid, zinc pyrithicone, sulfur, coal tar, or selenium sulfide. And continue to condition; dandruff shampoos do help the scalp but they can also dry out your hair.

ECZEMA RELIEF

If you have red, flaky patches on your scalp, you likely have eczema. However, because there are many kinds of eczema, and because your eczema could actually be psoriasis—a chronic, genetic condition that looks and feels a lot like eczema— it's best to consult a dermatologist to determine your best care.

TEMPORARY HAIR LOSS

On average, it is normal to lose 100 hairs each day. Temporary hair loss can also occur after pregnancy, or as a result of stress, illness or medication, but in most cases, the hair will grow back. To speed up the process, you can try one of these treatments (check with your doctor for more information): topical minoxidil (known as Rogaine), cortisone (may be injected, applied topically, or taken orally), tretinoins (such as Retin-A), Puva (a psoriasis treatment found to help with hair loss), and zinc. Temporary hair loss may also occur as the result of braiding the hair too tight, which forms scar tissue.

HEREDITARY HAIR LOSS

This condition affects 10 percent of all women. There are many treatments available, but they do not always live up to their claims. Topical minoxidil (sold as Rogaine for women) can help hold onto the hair that you have, hair-thickening shampoos can improve the appearance and density of your thinning hair, and, in severe cases, hair transplants may help. But, if you know thinning hair runs in your family, you'd be smart to start eating proactively too. Protein, sulfur-rich foods, flaxseed oil, vitamins A, B and C, wheat germ oil, gourd seed oil, cayenne pepper and ginger have all been shown to help build up the hair and keep the scalp healthy.

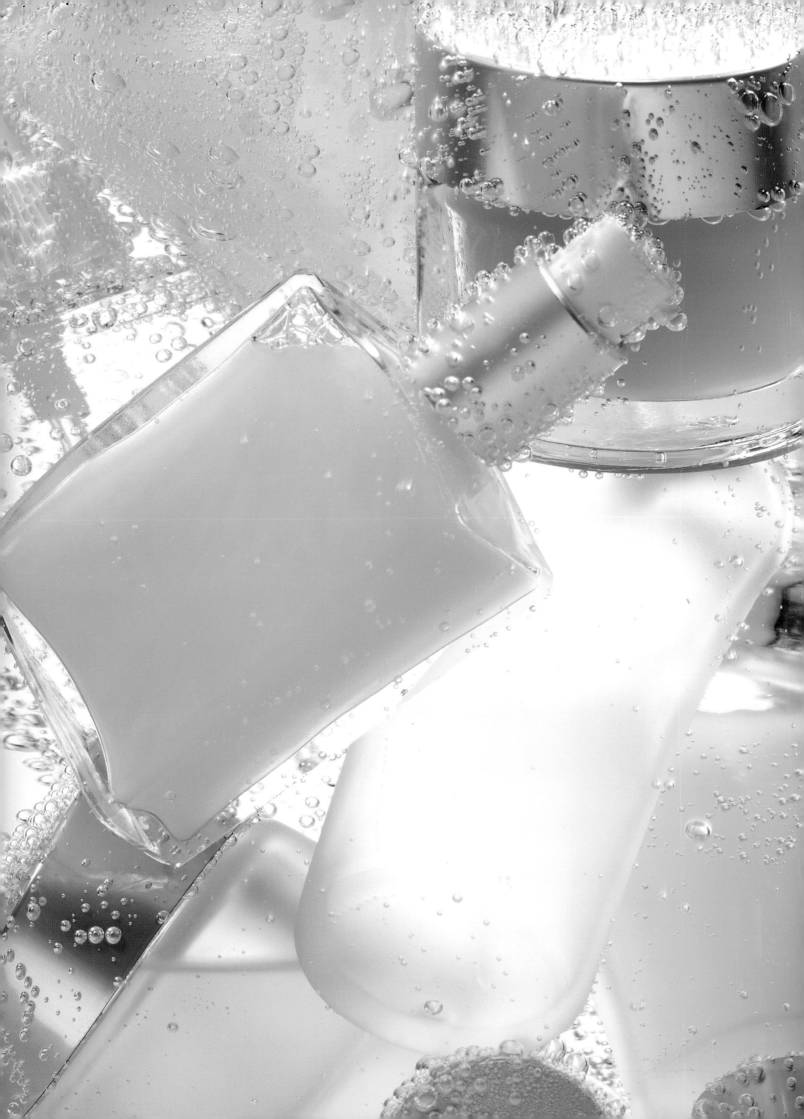

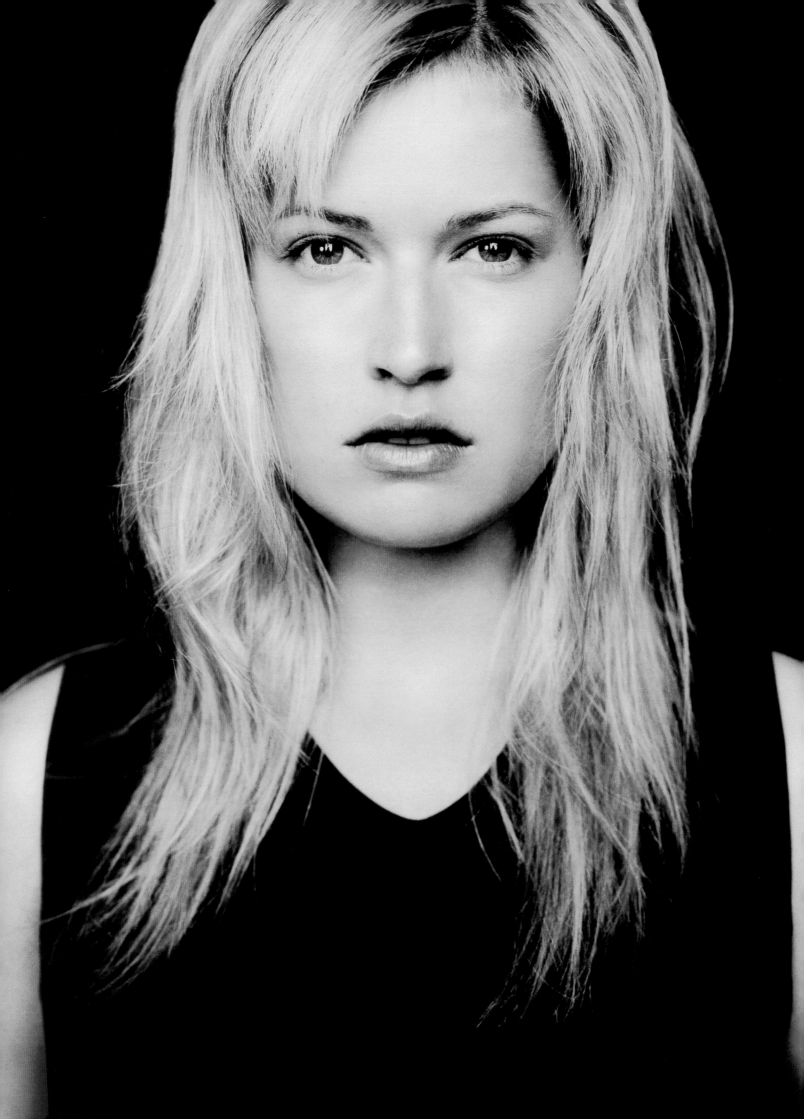

PREGNANCY

Hormonal changes during pregnancy will affect skin and hair. For the first three months, sebaceous glands can be overactive, leading to oily hair, so use mild shampoo daily. Thereafter, hair has a prolonged growth period, so it appears thicker and shinier. Avoid excessive chemical processing now. After the birth, as hormones readapt, hair can seem dull and hair loss excessive, but this is just hair that would have been lost earlier. It will grow back.

FRIZZY HAIR

Atmospheric moisture can be a nightmare, turning the sleekest locks into a frizzy mess. To overcome this, look for styling products that repel moisture—gloss, serums, styling creams and pomades containing silicones are good choices. Alternatively, try using a leave-in conditioner after shampooing. It won't overload the hair but will help retain moisture and prevent unwanted frizz.

STATICKY HAIR

All strands of hair have an electrical charge that is positive or negative. When either two positive or two negative hair strands repel each other, you'll get flyaways. This can occur as a result of the friction created when brushing or blow-drying the hair, or when you pull an item of clothing on over your head. Conditioners, mousse and styling sprays can help to restore the electrical balance, keeping your hair soft and static-free. If you are looking for a quick way to tame staticky hair, apply a fine mist of hairspray to your hairbrush or comb, then gently run it through flyaway hair.

OILY HAIR

Taking medication, stress, poor diet and hormonal imbalances can throw your scalp's oil-producing glands into a state of flux. The best way to combat greasiness is to wash every day with a gentle shampoo, then apply a light conditioner to just your ends. If you don't have time to shampoo, a dry shampoo—or even baby powder—applied at the roots will also help sop up excess oil.

DULL HAIR

This can result from bad circulation, buildup of styling products, harsh shampoos or poor diet. To make your hair appear more lustrous, stylists recommend smoothing on a glossing serum, then running a large clean fluffy makeup brush down the hair shaft to smooth the cuticles and give your hair a polished finish. For curly hair, a leave-in conditioner or conditioning spray applied before styling can help the cuticle lie flatter and reflect more light.

UNDER ATTACK

SUN EXPOSURE

Ultraviolet rays damage the hair, alter its color and can burn the scalp. To strengthen the hair and make it more resilient to UV attack, use hair-care products and stylers that contain UV protectors—look for those with Parsol 1789 (a UV filter). Or, in a pinch, use regular sunscreen on your scalp. Wearing a hat is also one of the safest ways to protect the hair and scalp, and can reduce the risk of heatstroke. During the summer or after sun exposure, hair will become drier and more susceptible to damage. To keep up its moisture content, swap your regular shampoo for a moisturizing formula. Unless your hair is extremely dry, it is not advisable to change to a moisturizing conditioner, which can overload the hair, making it look dull and lank. Instead, treat dry and brittle hair with a more intensive treatment once a week. Cut back on the use of heat-styling appliances during the summer to help maintain your hair's condition, and let it dry naturally. The warmth of the summer air will speed up the drying process; hair will be 75 percent dry in about fifteen minutes. To finish, use a hair dryer on a cool setting. When you are in the sun, don't pull your hair up into a topknot, as this exposes the ends of the hair to the sun's harmful rays. Instead, sweep your hair back to the nape of the neck, thus shielding your skin from the sun and hiding your ends, which are susceptible to damage.

WATER IRRITATION

The chemicals and impurities in chlorinated and salt water can ruin both the color and condition of the hair. If you have dry, damaged or color-treated hair, it is advisable to use a water-resistant hair-protection product before you go swimming. If you swim in chlorinated or salt water, you should always wash your hair as soon as you come out. After swimming in the ocean, if there is no alternative, you can rinse your hair with carbonated mineral water.

POLLUTION PERILS

Smoke, city grime and other pollutants can collect on the hair, making it look dull and lifeless. Other byproducts from cigarette smoke and natural gas can also discolor the hair—they are said to give white hair a yellowish tone. To remove such buildup, use a clarifying shampoo, which contains a high concentration of cleansers to remove stubborn dirt and ensure that there are no mineral residues left on the hair. If you find your hair smells of smoke or unpleasant cooking odors and you don't have time to wash it, spray a fine mist of perfume onto your comb or brush and run it through your hair.

WEATHER EXTREMES

Just as the wind, central heating and air conditioning have a drying effect on the skin, they can also damage the hair, making it very brittle. You should use a more intensive conditioner or a leave-in conditioner to combat dryness caused by cold weather. In freezing temperatures the hair picks up static electricity, making it hard to handle. You can reduce the static charge by spraying a hairbrush or comb with hairspray and gently running it through the hair. Central heating draws moisture from the hair and the scalp, which can also result in static. To reduce the drying effects of central heating, place large bowls of water near your radiators or use humidifiers. If you are in the snow, remember that the sun's rays are intensified by the reflection of the snow, so don't forget your hat!

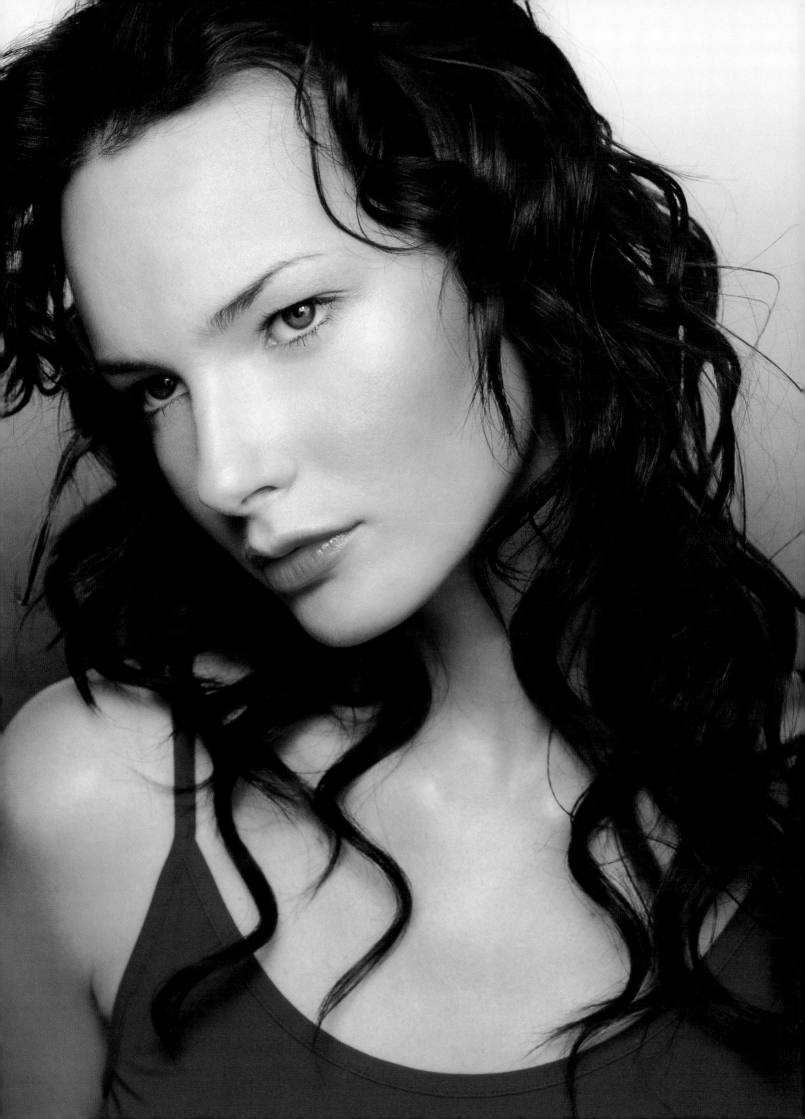

HAIRCYCLE

GROWTH PHASES

Hair grows about half an inch a month, and each strand has three growth phases before being replaced by a new hair. If not cut, hair strands will grow to 42 inches before being shed. Over time, growth decreases. To maintain healthy growth, massage the scalp regularly in order to stimulate the flow of nutrients, oxygen and blood to the hair follicles.

TEXTURE TURNS

It is inevitable that our hair's texture will change with age. The great body and volume that we experienced during adolescence will start to diminish and hair will become thinner and finer as it loses a third of its original diameter. However, clever cutting techniques and body-building stylers mean none of this should pose a serious problem.

COLOR CHANGES

As we age, hair loses its natural color: blonde hair fades, red hair picks up brown undertones and brunettes lose their natural highlights. This is because the activity of the hair's color-producing cells decreases and eventually stops over time (sometimes early in life), leaving you with white strands.

CONDITION ISSUE

The overall condition of the hair will change with time. When you're young, the sebaceous glands will be at their most active, but the production of the hair's natural oils slows down over time, causing hair to feel drier and coarser. To overcome this, step up the use of conditioning products and use a deep conditioner once a week.

adapt your hair-care regimen to suit your age

STRESS OUT

Work-related stress takes its toll on the hair and scalp. This can start during your twenties and will manifest itself through a dry, flaky scalp or the appearance of bald patches, which usually regrow. If you lead a stressful life, up your intake of B vitamins, found in wholegrain cereals, oily fish, yeast extracts, peas, natural yogurt, eggs and milk.

HAIR FOOD

Current research has shown that a fat-free diet can affect the condition of your hair, causing it to look dull and lifeless, and can also result in a dry scalp. If your hair suddenly becomes dry, it is advisable to increase your intake of essential fatty acids. These can be found in vegetable oils, in nuts and in oily fish, such as sardines and salmon.

FRAME WORK

As you get older, if you wear glasses, choose frames and a hairstyle that complement each other. Always take your glasses to the salon, so your hairdresser can see what you look like with them on. Remember, large glasses will seem out of place with super-short crops, while thin-framed, small glasses will seem unbalanced with masses of curls.

HORMONAL CHANGES

Our hormones play a vital role in the condition of our hair. Women may experience temporary hair loss while taking or coming off the Pill and those on HRT may notice an improvement in the hair's texture and condition. During pregnancy, hair will become drier, as increased estrogen production decreases sebum levels, but will look thicker.

BEAUTY INTELLIGENCE

Don't be fooled into thinking shampoos and conditioners loaded with vitamins are better for your hair—with the exception of B5, they can't be absorbed.

Get some extra mileage from your shampoo when you are on the move by using it to wash your body and even your clothes, too.

Normal hair should be able to stretch up to 30 percent of its length before breaking. Healthy hair will grow an average of six inches each year.

Brush tangled hair from the ends, working your way slowly to the roots, or you will have knots throughout. Work gently to avoid ripping the hair.

If the skin on your knees and elbows is dry but you have no moisturizer on hand, massage a small amount of creamy hair conditioner into the skin instead.

Condition dry, damaged hair by applying a protein deep conditioner, then blasting with a hair dryer. Heat helps the active ingredients work more effectively.

6

7

Rinsing with booze can improve the appearance of your hair. Beer will add shine, champagne can bring out blonde highlights and club soda can cut buildup.

If your hair feels rough when you finish shampooing, this could be an indication that the shampoo you are using is too harsh and not suitable for your hair type.

If you have colored hair, you should avoid using anti-dandruff shampoos, as these have been found to accelerate fading in some instances.

8

If you have fine hair, use a volumizing spray with polymers before blow drying. The heat will swell the polymers, making the hair appear thicker.

9

10

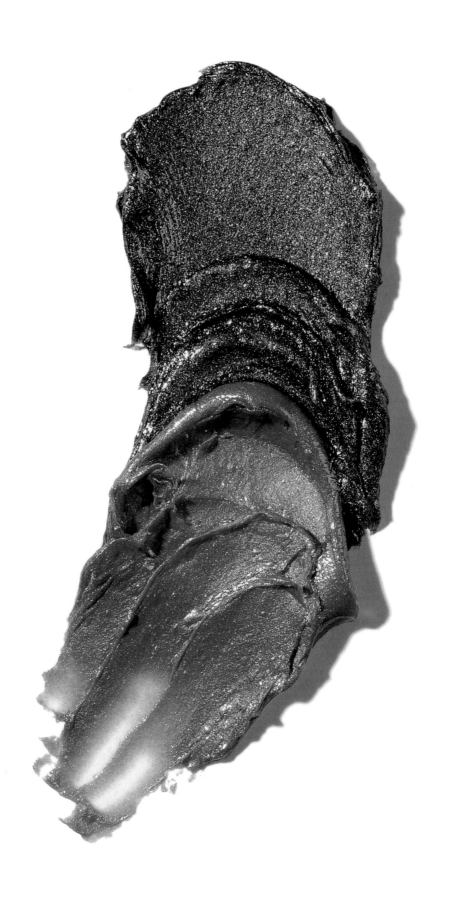

prep work

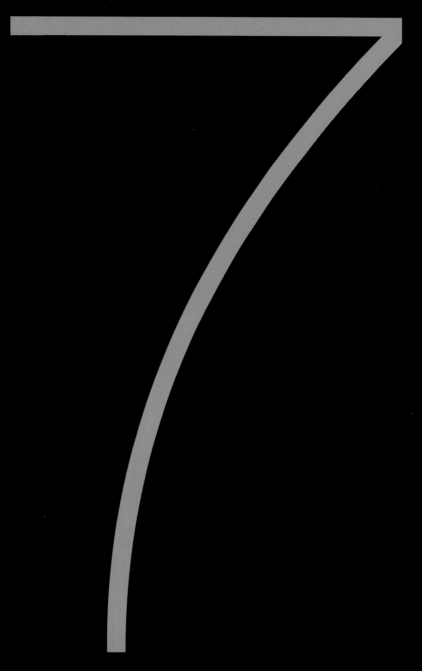

If you choose a haircut that complements the shape of your face, find styling products that suit your hair type, and use the right styling tools, there is no reason why every day can't be a good hair day. Here you'll find everything you need to know for your tress type.

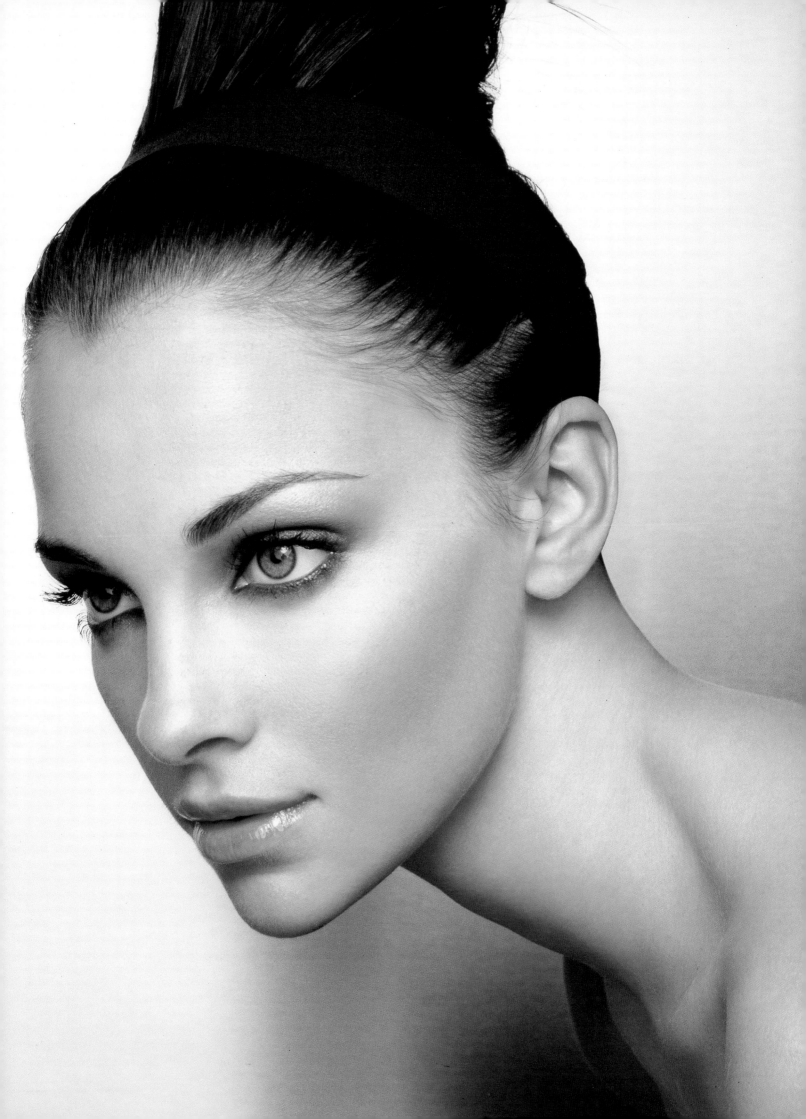

STYLING ESSENTIALS

WAX

is ideal for adding texture to short styles and definition to curly hair. To tame unruly hairs around the face or to redefine curls, look for a lightweight formula. Use a heavier wax on shorter styles or to break up thick hair. Apply sparingly, rubbing a small amount into the palms of your hands and then running them through your hair. Never apply wax to roots or fine hair.

MOUSSE

gives body to most styles, but works best on fine hair, creating hold without stickiness. For root lift, apply to your palms, rub together and massage into the roots before blow drying. To add body, apply from mid-shaft down, comb through and blow dry. For more hold, buy a formulation with extra holding properties.

STYLING CREME

can be applied to wet or dry hair to give it a smooth, flat finish. Some leave-in conditioners—those with stronger holding ingredients—double as styling creme (this is usually indicated on the package). Styling creme is ideal for extra dry or curly hair, which requires a lot of moisture. Use sparingly, about a dime-size drop, steering clear of roots.

HAIRSPRAY

is used as a finishing touch to
keep hair in place. Shake the can well
and then spray on, holding it at least six
inches from your head. Apply sparingly,
as too much can weigh the hair down.
For a post-styling fix to smooth flyaways, spray a brush or comb with
a fine mist of hairspray and then run it
through your hair. Avoid using
sprays containing alcohol if
you have dry hair.

SERUM

is usually silicone-based and forms
a microscopic film on the surface of the
hair shaft to enhance shine and softness.
Apply sparingly—two or three drops are
enough—or hair can look greasy. Use on
wet hair to deal with tangles or scrunch
into curls to reduce frizz and combat
static, or smooth down the hair shaft
to tame unruly cuticles and temporarily
seal split ends.

POMADE

is softer than wax and does not
weigh the hair down so much. Use to
slick hair back, smooth cuticles and add
definition to short styles. Apply sparingly
and avoid altogether if you have fine hair.
Anti-humectant pomades help prevent
hair from getting frizzy in humid
conditions, forming a moisture-repellent
shield on the hair shaft.

GEL

is available in different consistencies,
ranging from lightweight sprays to thicker
jelly types. Use on wet hair to protect
before blow drying and add volume, or
on dry styles to slick the hair back or to
add texture to shorter styles. If gel dries
on the hair and feels brittle, mix with a
small amount of serum before applying.

BRUSH WORK

Brushing your hair will help smooth the cuticles, enhancing shine, stimulate the blood supply to hair follicles, promoting healthy growth, and remove accumlated dirt and dead skin cells. Always brush your hair before shampooing to make it tangle-free. Forget anything you might have been told about the need to brush your hair 100 strokes a day before you go to bed—in fact, over-zealous brushing can tear the hair and is likely to strip it of all its natural oils.

BRISTLE CHOICE

Choose a hairbrush to suit your particular hair type and styling requirements. Brushes with natural bristles are less damaging to the hair, but natural bristles alone will be too soft to penetrate thick hair, which needs the added strength supplied by a mix of nylon and natural bristles. For thick, curly hair, a brush with closely spaced, all-nylon bristles will offer maximum control for smoothing or straightening; widely spaced bristles will minimize pull to enhance wave and volume. For fine or thinning hair, use a soft-bristle brush. For African-American hair that has been relaxed, use a natural-bristle brush, and on curly styles use a wide-toothed comb.

THE RIGHT BRUSH

Flat brushes, usually oval or rectangular in shape, are ideal for smoothing and detangling the hair. Paddle brushes have oversized, flat bases, making them suitable for longer hair. Vent brushes have vented, hollow centers to allow a heated stream of air to flow through the brush and the hair, which ensures high-speed drying and added volume to almost any style. They are especially good for blow-drying relaxed hair. For straightening curly hair, smoothing sleeker styles or styling short hair, round brushes are best. For curling, the smaller the cylinder of the brush, the tighter the curl. If you have baby-fine hair or pieces that are very short as a result of breakage or chemical processing, you should use a small round brush and a hair dryer to blend them in with the rest of your hair. For straightening, smaller brushes—three to four inches in diameter—are suitable for shorter styles, while brushes with a larger diameter should be used on longer hair. To speed up the drying process, try a round brush with bristles embedded in a metal or aluminium barrel, as this will heat up when it is used with a hair dryer and help to set your style.

EXPERT ADVICE

If you love brushing your hair vigorously, to make sure that you do as little damage as possible, work through your hair first with a comb to deal with any tangles before you use your hairbrush. Always brush your hair gently, trying not to pull or twist it too much. Do not brush your hair when it is wet, as it will be water-logged and weak then and susceptible to damage. Hairdressers advise not to brush your hair until it is at least 80 percent dry for the best results when styling.

UPKEEP

Brushes should be washed at regular intervals with hot, soapy water. To deal with the buildup of hair on a brush, run your comb vertically between the rows of bristles to loosen the hairs and then ease them out with your fingers. Throw away brushes and combs with broken bristles or teeth, as these can tear and snag the hair and also scratch the scalp.

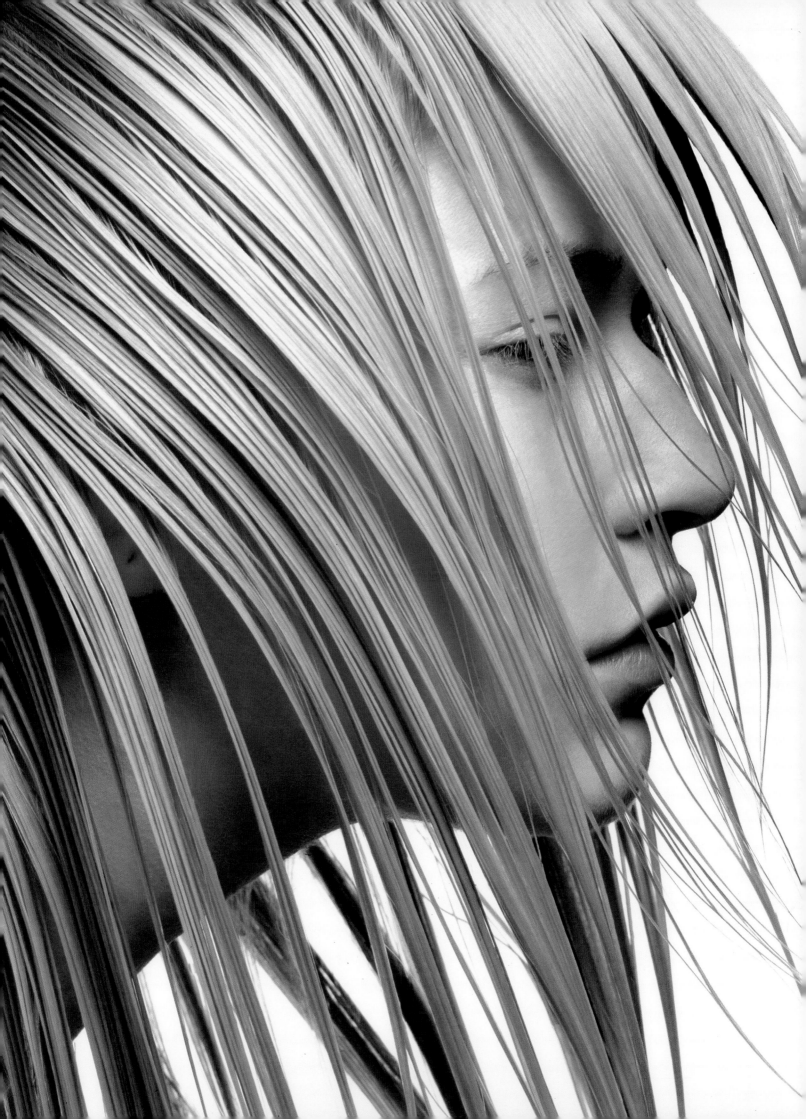

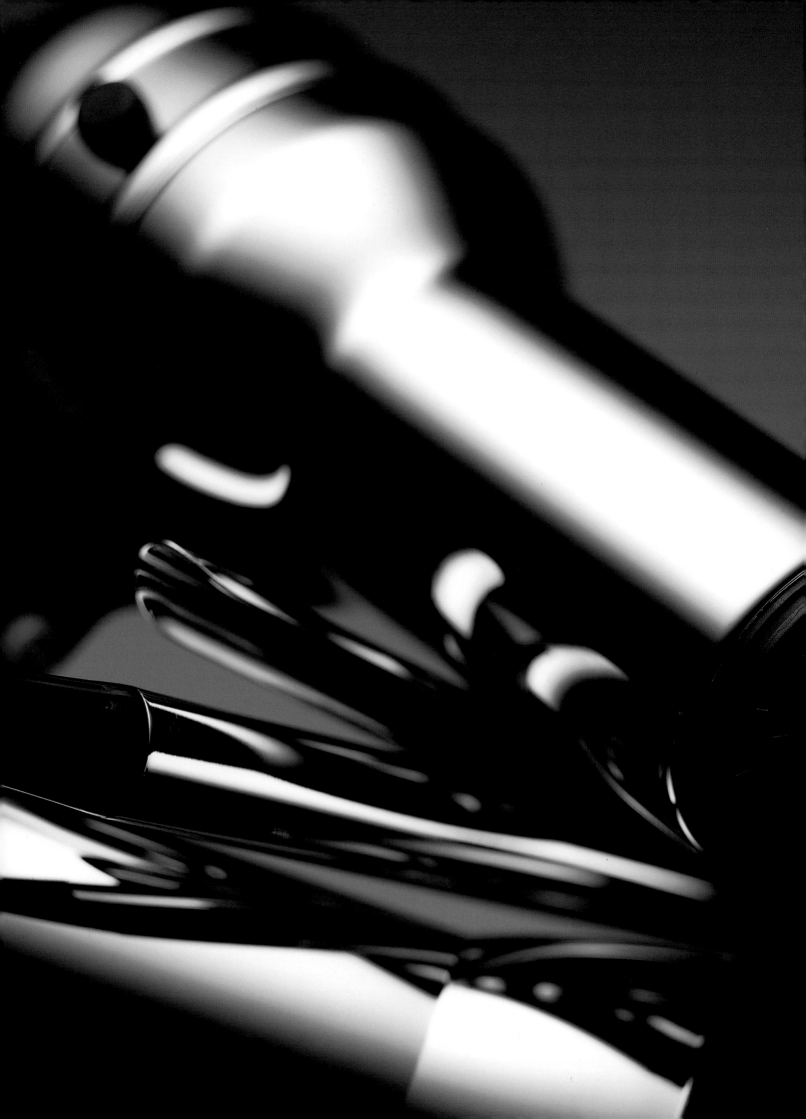

STYLING APPLIANCES

Whatever style you might want to achieve is possible with the help of the latest heated appliances. The only drawback is that heat can damage the hair, but you can always overcome this by using a heat-protectant styling product.

HAIR DRYER
Look for a hair dryer with at least two speeds and three settings—cool, medium and hot. The heat from a hair dryer can reach 300 degrees Fahrenheit, which is as hot as an oven. Dry your hair on warm, and use hot air only at the end for setting your style. Look for a 1,600+ watt dryer. Hair dryers last on average between 200 and 300 hours. Never use a dryer without the filter in place, otherwise hair strands can get singed. Clean the filter regularly, as a blocked filter will cause the dryer to overheat. You should never wrap the dryer's cord tightly around it. If you have curly or permed hair, use a diffuser—a plastic or cloth attachment that fits on the end of the nozzle of the dryer—while blow drying. This will gently spread the airflow over your hair without disturbing the curl. For the best results, switch back and forth between the low and medium settings, while cupping the hair in the palm of your hand.

CURLING IRON
This is a great device for creating curls at high speed. Choose your iron based on the type of curl you want to create, remembering that the diameter of the barrel will dictate the size of the curl. If you want to see movement right up to the roots, place a comb next to the scalp before you wind the barrel up the hair shaft to the roots. This will form a barrier to protect you from burning your scalp. To clean the iron, you should wipe with it a damp cloth once cooled.

HEATED CURLERS
You can set your hair in ten minutes with heated curlers. They make restyling the hair a breeze. The secret is to remove the curlers when they have cooled and the hair is completely cool, otherwise the movement created will drop. While heated curlers make dealing with unruly bangs and bed-head quick and easy, you should never use them on wet hair.

STRAIGHTENING IRONS
Using a high dose of heat, these literally flatten the hair, so apply a heat-protectant spray first to reduce damage. Use only intermittently, and never on wet or damp hair.

CRIMPERS
If you want to create waves in the hair, try using crimpers. They often come with a range of attachments to help you achieve different waves or even to straighten the hair. Use only on dry hair and avoid altogether if you have bleached hair, as the high levels of heat generated will dry the hair and this could result in breakage.

YOUR BEST CUT

If you're planning a drastic change or want to use your hairstyle to make the most of your features, talk to your hairdresser first to get a good understanding of what can be achieved. There are always ways to disguise features that you dislike and play up your strengths.

FRINGE BENEFITS

If you have a high, low or uneven hairline, disguise it with bangs. To draw attention away from thinning hair around the hairline, opt for bangs that are tapered down the temples. The longer the bangs, the wider the face will appear. A round face needs short bangs to elongate it. Wide, broad bangs can make the eyes appear larger, but can also make the face look wider. If you have a high forehead, disguise it with long bangs, and if you have a low forehead, choose a style with wispy rather than full bangs.

ROUND FACE

To flatter a round face, find a style that both adds height at the crown and retains overall length. Styles that are razor-cut at the sides soften your look and narrow the face. Shorter bangs with a blunt finish look good. Avoid bobs, extremely flat or curly styles and center parts, as they accentuate the face's shape.

SQUARE FACE

Soften an angular face and strong jawline with a feminine cut. Opt for longer styles with casual layers or curls, bangs that skim the top of the eyebrows to balance the proportions of the face, or a side part. Avoid sharp, jaw-length cuts, square, heavy bangs or styles that are cropped at the nape. Remember that symmetrical and geometric shapes will only emphasize your face's angularity.

LONG FACE

To balance a long face, experiment with bangs that are cut wide to give the illusion of width at the temples, and opt for a chin-length cut, which will add width around the lower face. You should avoid long, straight styles, one-length cuts and styles without bangs, as these will make the shape of your face more pronounced.

OVAL FACE

This face shape is easy for hairdressers to work with because almost all hairstyles will work. Oval faces do have a tendency to be wider at the forehead; if you feel this is too apparent, opt for bangs.

HEART-SHAPED FACE

Find a style that will add height at the crown and width around the jawline and chin. Graduated layers are always a flattering option for this face shape. Avoid a center part, as this will emphasize the point of your chin. Try a high, off-center part instead.

JAWLINE

Hairdressers maintain that the distance and angle between your chin and your earlobe should determine the length of your hair. If the distance is short, and you have a good jawline, any length will suit your face. If, however, you have a long, sloping jawline, you should avoid very short hairstyles and tightly pulled-back looks.

IRREGULAR FEATURES

If you have a very pointed chin, choose a hairstyle that adds width at the jawline to draw attention away from it. If you have a weak chin, wear your hair so the ends skim the sides of your chin. Slim down a broad neck by tucking your hair behind your ears and letting it fall softly around your neck. If you have a prominent nose, a soft layered style will be the most flattering.

CUTTING TECHNIQUES

If your hair is fine and flyaway, opt for a short, layered cut, which is easy to manage and will create the illusion of body. For the best results, layers of different lengths should be cut into the hair. If your hair is thick, frizzy and hard to handle, avoid a lot of layers. Opt instead for graduated layers around the base of your hair, which will help weigh the hair down and add softness.

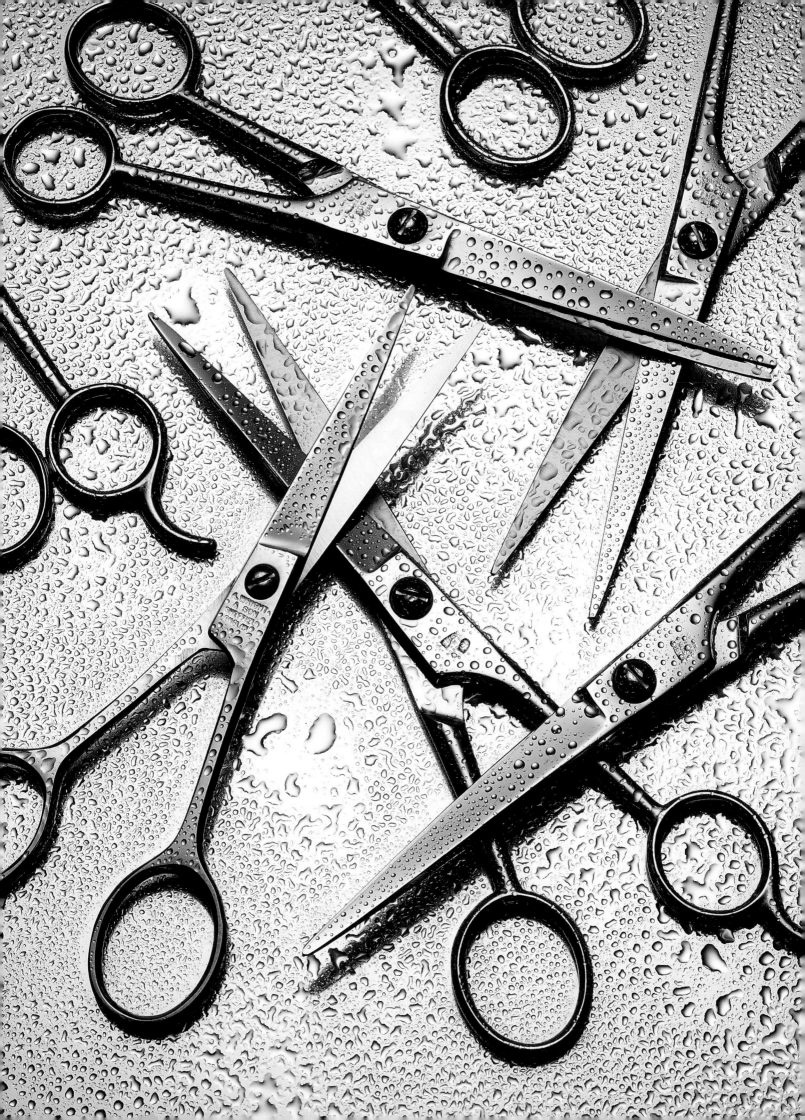

HAIRSOLUTIONS

REGULAR CUTS

Most stylists recommend that you get your hair cut every six weeks. While this will not make your hair grow any faster, it will keep it in good condition. Investing in a good haircut pays off—as your hair grows, the style will continue to look well-groomed. Request a consultation with a stylist before deciding on any haircut—most salons offer this service free.

SPLIT ENDS

Slathering on different products won't repair split ends. The only way to get rid of them is to have your hair cut, although regular trims can help prevent the problem. To temporarily seal split ends, massage a styling creme, wax, serum or even a bit of Vaseline into them.

PRODUCT BUILDUP

If you use gels, mousses or sprays daily, your hair can end up looking limp due to residue buildup. To remedy, use a clarifying shampoo once a week. To increase the product's efficiency, apply it to your hair while it is dry, before stepping into the shower, so as not to dilute it.

DOUBLE-DUTY 'DO

A creamy conditioner will double as a styling aid when mixed with an equal amount of hair gel. Apply to short-to-medium hair and mold in place. Rinse your hair at the end of the day to reveal shiny, healthy locks.

follow these simple steps for healthy hair

CONDITION TIP
Leaving conditioners on for more than the time specified will not boost their effectiveness. Most conditioners only coat the hair, so they will be as effective after one minute as after fifteen. However, oil or panthenol-based deep-conditioning treatments do penetrate the hair shaft, which is why they need to be left on longer for maximum benefits.

GET A GRIP
Glass and plastic shampoo and conditioner bottles that twist open can be a challenge when your hands are wet. To remedy this problem, wrap a few rubber bands around the top so you have something to grasp.

HEAT CHECK
If you have greasy hair, always use your hair dryer on the cool setting, as the hot air can activate your oil glands and increase sebum production. Using a hair dryer on a cool setting also benefits your style, since unnecessary heat on the scalp makes it perspire, which can cause your style to droop and lost its shape.

GEL REVIVER
If you've slicked your hair back with gel and it starts to lose its shape and definition, you shouldn't add more product, as this could overload the hair, making it look dull and lifeless. Take a tip from the experts: wet your fingertips and run them through your hair to resculpt and revitalize it. Or, brush your hair to remove the gel and start from scratch.

BEAUTY INTELLIGENCE

1 Flip your head forward when brushing to speed blood flow to the scalp and also to get better lift at the roots.

2 Try to hold your hair dryer above and behind your head, like your hairdresser would do. The hot air will then flow down the hair shaft and seal the cuticles.

3 Don't worry if you don't have time to shampoo every day. The natural oils in unwashed hair make it much easier to control and style.

4 Scrunch equal amounts of hair gel and serum into curls. Serum will stop the gel from stiffening as it dries, stop curls from frizzing and boost shine.

5 Don't try running a brush through curled hair. Instead, use your fingers to break up the curls, otherwise you'll end up with a frizzy mess.

To give dull, lifeless-looking hair a quick shine, spread serum from mid-shaft to ends using a fluffy powder brush.

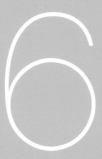

If you have sensitive eyes, try using baby shampoo. This will clean your hair as well as regular shampoo—minus the irritation.

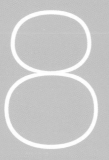

Hair serum, which can be used to protect and to polish tresses, can also be smoothed onto bare legs in the summer to give skin a more radiant finish.

You can massage styling wax into nail cuticles to hydrate and protect them. If the wax is hard, gently heat it with a hair dryer first to make it easier to apply.

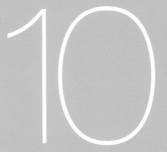

Try not to keep touching your hair once it has been styled; otherwise, it can lose its shape and body and become greasy.

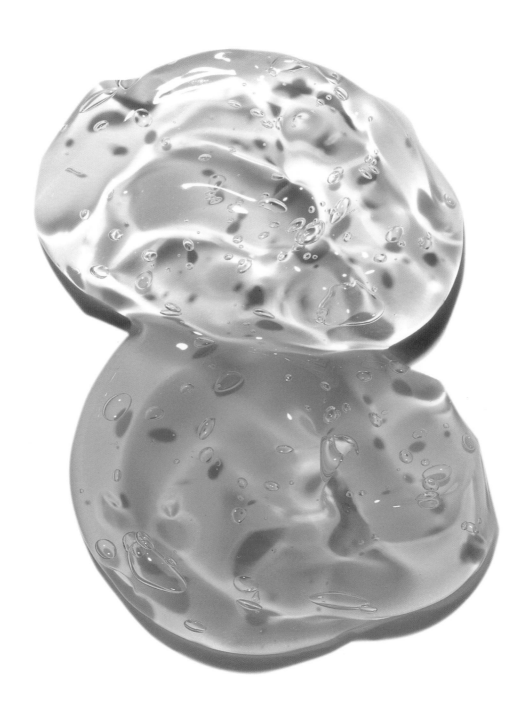

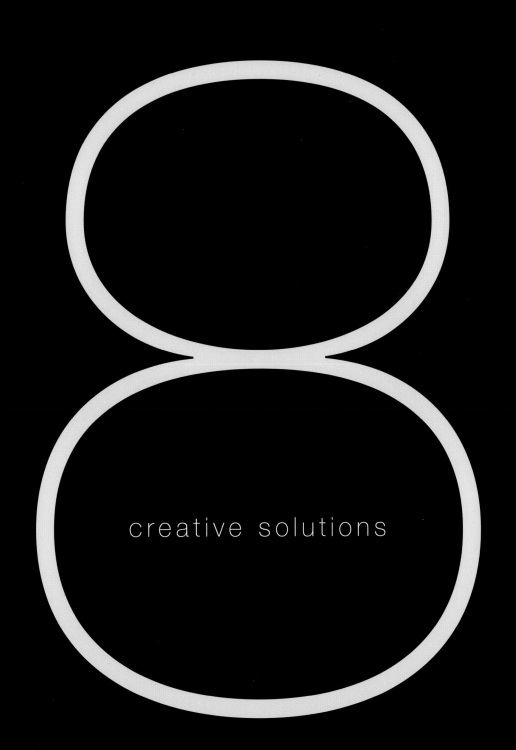

creative solutions

Hairstyling can be done quickly with minimum fuss as long as you know how. Whether you want to create curls, wear your hair up or let it hang loose, the aim is to look sexy and modern—but never overdone. Your goal should be to find a hairstyle you can create effortlessly in a few minutes.

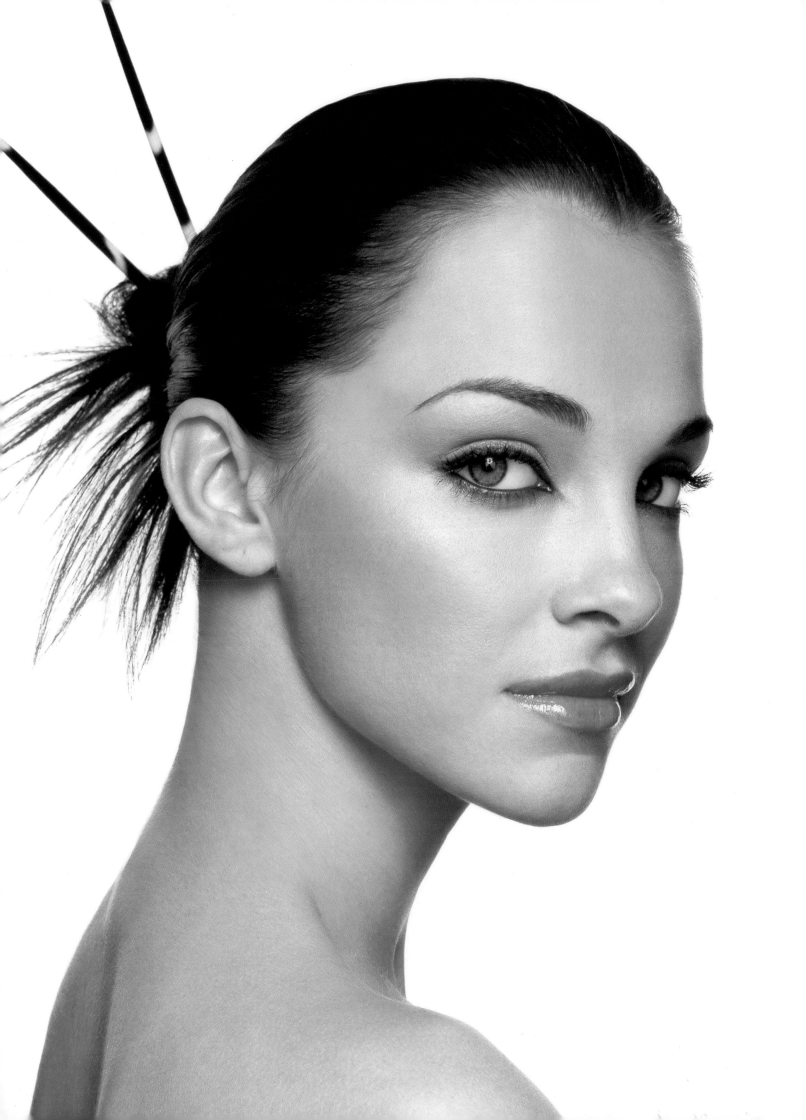

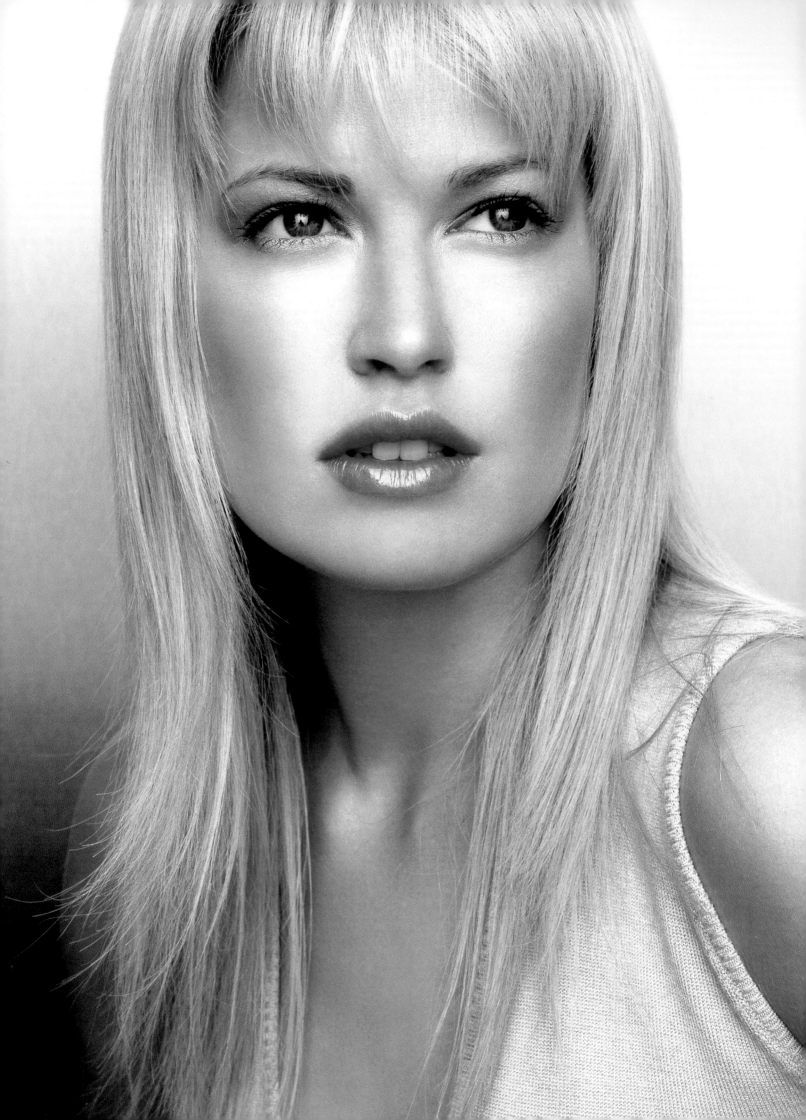

BLOW DRYING

PREP WORK Before blow drying, use a wide-toothed comb to remove all tangles. Apply a heat-styling aid to protect the hair and comb through in the direction and shape of the finished style. Start off by blow drying the hair all over, using your fingers to shake out excess moisture. Then, blow dry the under sections with a natural-bristle brush, making sure that each one is completely dry before moving on to the next, and gradually work up the head. Hot hair can feel damp, so give your hair a cool blast of air before you decide whether it is really dry or not.

STYLING ADVICE Styling your hair when it is wet can be damaging. Instead, blow or air dry until it is 50–60 percent dry if curly or wavy and 80 percent if straight. The more styling your hair needs, the damper it should be when you start.

DRYING TECHNIQUES You should always move the dryer back and forth over your hair, even when you are concentrating on one particular section. Either work in small rotating motions or gently shake the dryer, as holding heat on one spot will dry the hair out and could burn the scalp.

HEAT CONTROL Do not use a dryer on the hottest setting when you are working on the roots, as this could burn the scalp—and also flatten the hair. Moderate heat (or slightly hotter for frizzy or thick hair) will help create volume. If your hair is fine, always work with the dryer on a cool to moderate setting to prevent it from frying.

KEEP COOL If you are using a brush while blow drying to curl or style your hair, allow each section of hair to cool before removing the brush, otherwise the shape you have created might droop. Alternatively, before removing the brush, blast the hair with the dryer on a cool setting to finish.

COWLICKS A cowlick is a small area of hair that sticks up around the hairline and does not grow in the same direction as the rest of the hair. To tame it, try using a round brush to blow dry the cowlick to one side first, then the other. This should straighten the cowlick out.

AIR FLOW Always aim the air flow of your hair-dryer down the hair shaft, to ensure that the cuticles lie flat and the hair looks shiny (if you point the air flow up the hair shaft, it will dishevel the cuticles and the hair will look dull and lifeless).

LIMITED TIME If you are pushed for time, start blow drying the hair around your face first, as this is what people really see, then work on the top sections. If time does not permit, allow the under sections to dry naturally. Or, comb wet hair into shape and then wait a bit; when nearly dry, use your hair dryer and a styling brush to finish.

TWIST

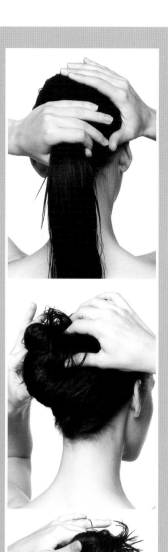

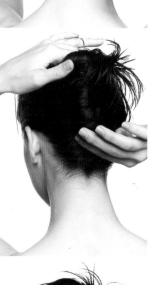

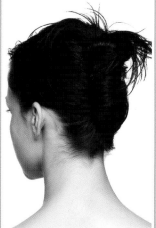

1. You don't need to be a hair pro to master this style. If you arm yourself with a comb and bobby pins, you can twist your hair up into an interesting shape in seconds. Gently comb through and pull it all back to the nape of your neck, as if creating a ponytail. Instead of securing with a band, twist the hair until it is taut, and then twist up the back of the head.

2. Secure in place with bobby pins where needed, but make sure the pins aren't visible. If you have problems seeing what you are doing, look into a wall mirror and then inspect your work with a hand-held mirror, holding it behind you.

3. If you find that stray hairs have popped out of the twist, use the pointed end of a comb to tuck them in, securing with extra pins.

4. This is a great style for you to create when your hair is still wet, because it will dry in place. It will also give the hair interesting movement and body when you take the pins out and unravel your hair.

PONYTAIL

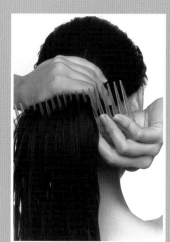

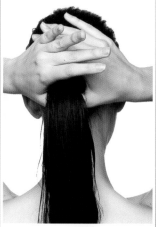

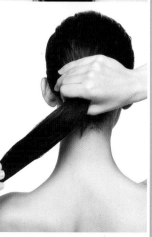

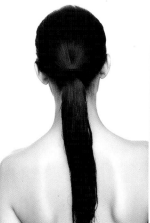

1. Anyone can achieve this look in four simple steps. Start by brushing the hair to make sure that it is completely tangle-free.

2. Then comb the hair back toward the nape of your neck, ensuring that it is tightly pulled by running your hands through it. This will tame unruly hairs and reduce static that may have occurred while combing.

3. Do not secure with a rubber band as it can snag and tear the hair and is difficult to remove. Look instead for special bands that are either fabric-covered or designed not to rip the hair.

4. Once in place, roughly divide your ponytail into two parts and draw them out vertically to tighten the tail. Comb through again for a sleek finish. For added interest, curl the ends of your hair or add extra shine by patting glossing serum over the hair that's pulled back.

CURLS

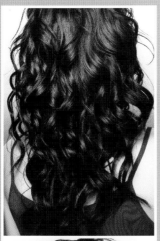

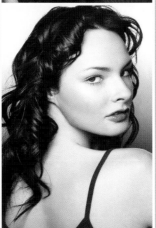

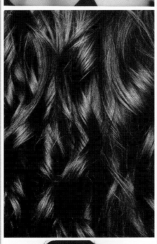

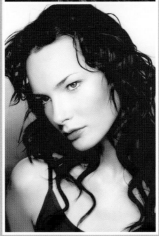

1. If you have a natural wave to your hair it will be easy to curl, while straight hair will need a little more work. Curl hair by setting it with curlers (use heated curlers on dry hair or Velcro curlers on damp hair). The type of curl created will be determined by the size of curlers used: the smaller the curlers, the tighter the curl. Large curlers will create rough-and-tumble, loose curls. Spray your hair with a sculpting or setting lotion before using curlers.

2. The angle at which you wind your curlers will determine the amount of root lift. So, if hair is wound around the curler at a 90-degree angle it will create maximum root lift, while 45 degrees will give minimum root lift.

3. Always wind hair around the curler from the ends up.

4. Do not remove curlers until hair is completely dry, or the body will simply drop out. To style curls, do not comb them through; use your fingers to separate them instead.

SLICKED BACK

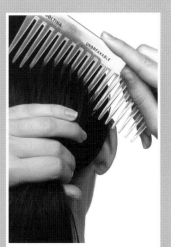

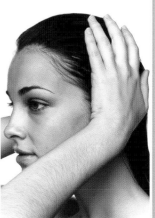

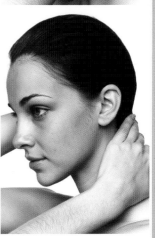

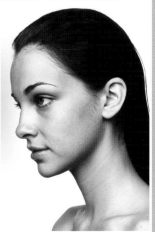

1. Slicking it back is one of the simplest and quickest ways to style the hair—and you can create either a high-shine, smooth finish or a more textured look. For a more natural-looking finish, use a minimal amount of hair mousse or gel and gently run a wide-toothed comb through dry or damp hair. For a sleeker finish, smooth wax or pomade on dry or damp hair and then comb in place. If you do not have gel, mousse or wax on hand, use an oil-based moisturizer to slick hair back instead.

2. Carefully work the comb through the hair to distribute the product evenly and then shape into the desired style. Using a wide-toothed comb will create a textured finish.

3. After combing, run your hands through your hair to tame strays and ensure a smooth finish. To keep in place, apply a fine mist of hairspray.

4. If you have long hair, you can slick it back and then go on to either secure it in a ponytail or pin it up.

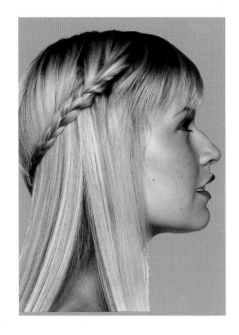

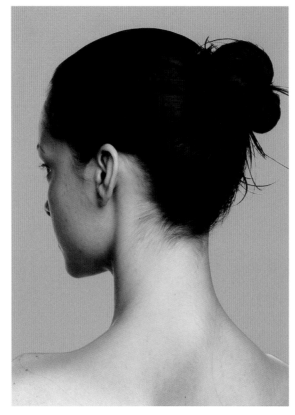

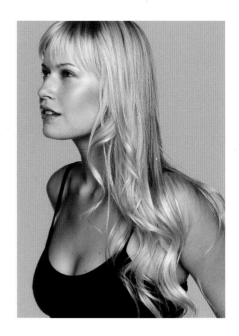

2

1

BRAID

If you are looking for a fun variation on
braids, you can simply braid
the front sections of your hair by each
temple and then pull them back
and secure them together with an elastic.
Let the rest of the hair hang straight down.
This is a great way to add interest
to a one-length style. If you are bored
with the traditional three-strand braid and
want to try something different, use just two
sections of hair and wind them around each
other. When you get to the ends of the hair,
secure the braids with an elastic.

TOPKNOT

Ensure hair is tangle-free, then comb
it toward the crown of the head and pull it
into a high ponytail. Secure with a ponytail
holder, then wrap the hair in a circular
motion around the tie in a bun shape.
Secure with bobby pins. For a modern
finish, splay the ends out and mold into
an interesting shape, then fix with a light
hairspray. You can also reposition the bun
at the nape of the neck or the middle
of the back of the head.

3

DROP CURLS

If you have shoulder-length or longer
hair that is straight or has a natural wave,
you can create an interesting finish by
curling from mid-shaft to your ends. Start at
the front with one-inch-wide sections of hair
and wrap them around a curling iron,
working from the mid-shaft to the end. Clasp
hair in the iron for thirty to sixty seconds,
depending on your hair type: fine hair will
absorb heat more quickly. Unravel, then
move on to the next section. If you're using
heated curlers, follow the same procedure
but wind hair from the ends up the hair shaft
until you reach the tops of the ears. Secure
in place and move on to the next section.

six secrets for easy hairstyling

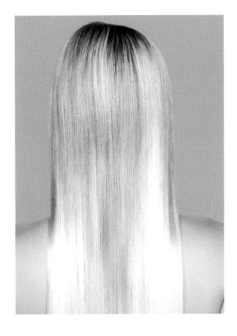

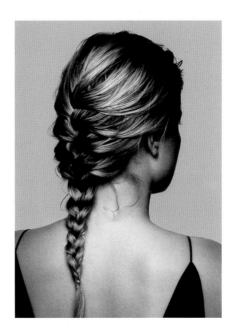

5

6

"FRENCH" BRAID

To successfully French braid the hair, comb through to remove tangles, then divide into three equal sections. Weave the left section over the middle section, then weave the right section over the middle section, repeating the process and folding in new hair from each side until you reach your ends. Secure with an elastic. Once you have finished, spritz the hair with a fine mist of hairspray to keep it in place. If you feel the total look is too neat, simply ease out a few strands of hair around the front. If you pull too much out by mistake, you don't need to start again from scratch. Using bobby pins, tuck the hair back into the braid and secure in place.

4

STRAIGHT

To get your hair pin-straight, first apply a smoothing cream, then comb it through and partially dry the hair, using your fingers to shake out excess moisture. Separate a one-inch section of hair from the nape with a comb and pin the rest of the hair out of the way. Using a round brush, dry this section. For the best results, glide the brush from roots to ends and direct the air flow from the hair dryer down the hair shaft, following the brush as you work. Make sure that each section is completely dry before you move on to the next one. Gradually proceed up the head, working in one-inch sections. After drying, you can run a straightening iron over any areas that still need smoothing—particularly your ends. Then smooth on a small amount of serum to give the hair a polished finish.

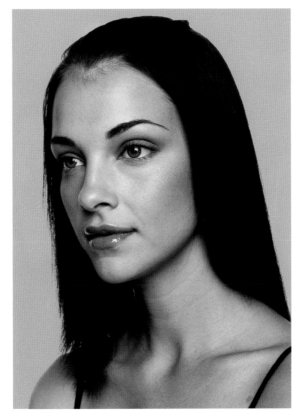

PULLED BACK

This look is ideal for one-length styles, longer hair with layers or if you are growing out your bangs The secret is to make sure the hair is absolutely straight and ultra-shiny. If you're not an expert at blow drying your hair straight, try using a heated straightening iron. Once hair is smooth, comb it off the face and make two parts (using the center of each iris as a guide) back to the crown. Secure this section with a hair comb so that hair is held neatly off the face.

STYLINGWORK

STYLE SAVERS

When you are traveling, it's always possible to get more mileage from your hairstyling appliances. When you are packing, wrap your necklaces around a Velcro curler and secure in place with a hair elastic. This will ensure that chains do not tangle and get knotted. Also, hair dyers can be used to dry lingerie and any other small items of clothing after washing.

LOCKS LOCK-DOWN

On a humid day, healthy hair can swell almost 15 percent. (Damaged hair fares even worse.) To minimize expansion—and frizz—finish off your style with a creamy product that contains silicone. The product's weight will help prevent puffiness better than a light hairspray or gel.

SATIN SLIP

If you always wake up with bed-head hair, try changing your pillowcase. Satin pillowcases allow the hair to slide across the pillow gently as you move in your sleep, whereas cotton causes friction and disrupts the hair. Using a satin pillowcase also means that you will not end up with crease marks on your face if you tend to sleep nuzzled into the pillow.

EASY CURLS

To curl hair with a natural wave, take random one- or two-inch sections of damp hair, twist tightly and literally scrunch up into small balls and secure in place. Let dry naturally, only unravelling when the hair is completely dry. To finish, do not comb through but tip your head upside down and use your fingers to break up the curl and enhance the movement created.

simple steps to successful hairstyling

ROOT LIFT

A foolproof way to achieve root lift that lasts is to work through the roots with a vent brush. While you are blow drying your hair, lift individual sections and blast them with air. You will also find that tipping your head upside down or leaning your head to one side as you blow dry will maximizing your hair's volume.

FLYAWAY HAIR

If you have a problem with staticky, flyaway hair, try using an anti-static clothes spray. You should never apply this directly to the hair, but can spray a small amount on to a comb or hairbrush and then gently run it through the hair. However, proceed with caution as overzealous combing or brushing is likely to result in more static.

STEAM STYLE

When you run a bath, close the bathroom door so the steam from the water doesn't evaporate, then spray your hair with setting lotion and put curlers in before getting into the bath. The steam will help set the curls. Remove the curlers when your hair is completely dry and run your fingers through the hair to break up the curls and to add definition.

THICKENING TREAT

If you have baby-fine blonde hair and want to make it look fuller and also appear lighter, hairdressers recommend using a dry shampoo. This will add body and make the hair easier to manage. Just remember, less is more, so try to be as light-handed as possible during application. To remove, simply brush the hair.

BEAUTY INTELLIGENCE

1

If you have coarse, dry hair, try adding jojoba oil to your styling regimen. It is similar in structure to the hair's natural oil, helping to hydrate and smooth.

2

Choose a hair dryer that is 1500 watts or more. If you use anything less, it will take too long to dry your hair, increasing the likelihood of damage.

3

After using hairspray, try not to brush your hair, otherwise you will remove all the product you have just applied. Instead, run a comb gently through your hair.

4

Apply conditioner to your hair at the beach to shield it from UV rays. The heat will also intensify the product's efficacy, so your hair will be extra soft.

5

If your locks look flat a few hours after styling, give them a boost by tipping your head down and running a brush through the undersides of your hair.

With age, hair becomes more fragile and susceptible to damage, so use a soft brush and keep chemical processing and heat-styling to a minimum.

6 Avoid over-brushing your hair. The "100 strokes a day" rule is from the 1900s, when women washed their hair far less often. Five to ten strokes should do it.

7 If your hair gets dry and brittle in the winter, indoor heating is a likely culprit. Humidifiers will increase the amount of water in the air—and in your hair.

8 To add interesting texture to dry hair without making it looking greasy or overloaded with product, use a small amount of leave-in conditioner.

9 If your tights get a snag, use a little hairspray to keep it from running. Do not be heavy-handed, though, or your tights might end up stuck to your legs.

10

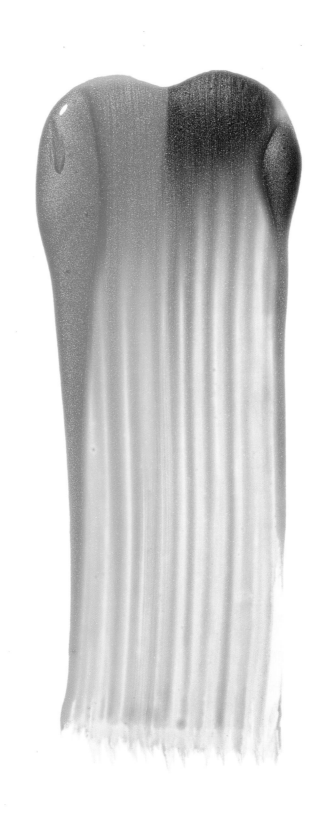

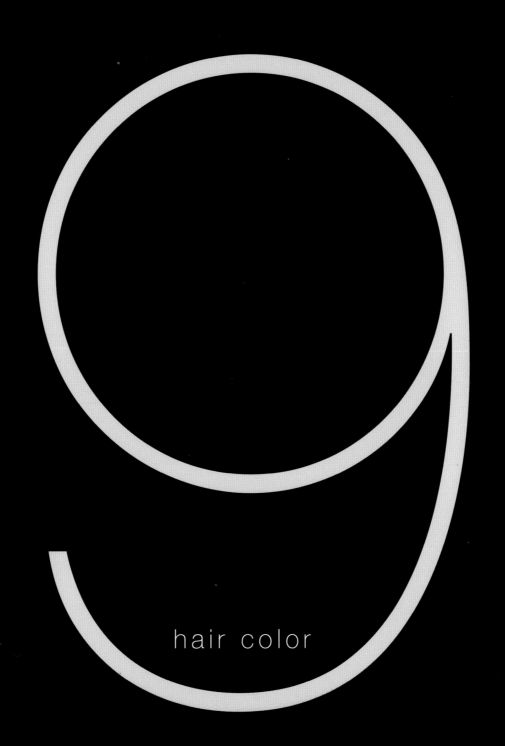

hair color

Whether you go for bold red, rich brown or glossy blonde, hair color can make a great impact on the way you look and feel. The new generation of colorants are enriched with conditioning ingredients, so if you want a drastic change or just subtle enhancement, you can achieve results without wreaking havoc on the overall health of your hair.

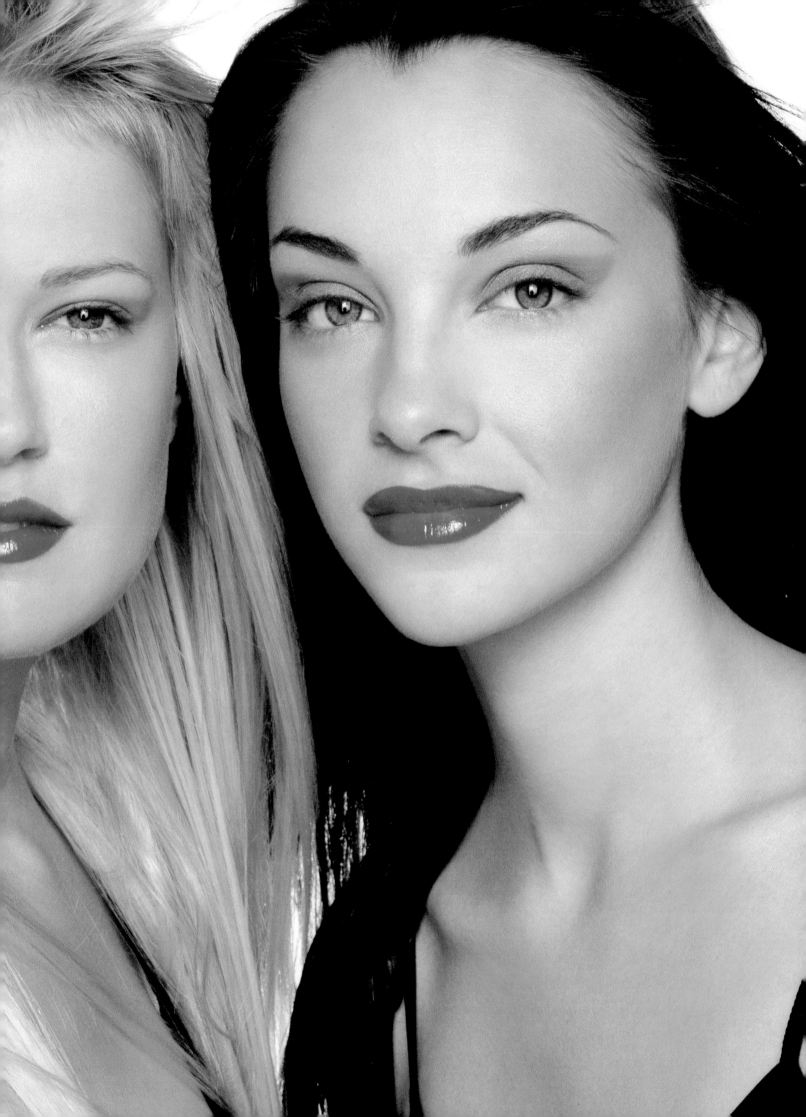

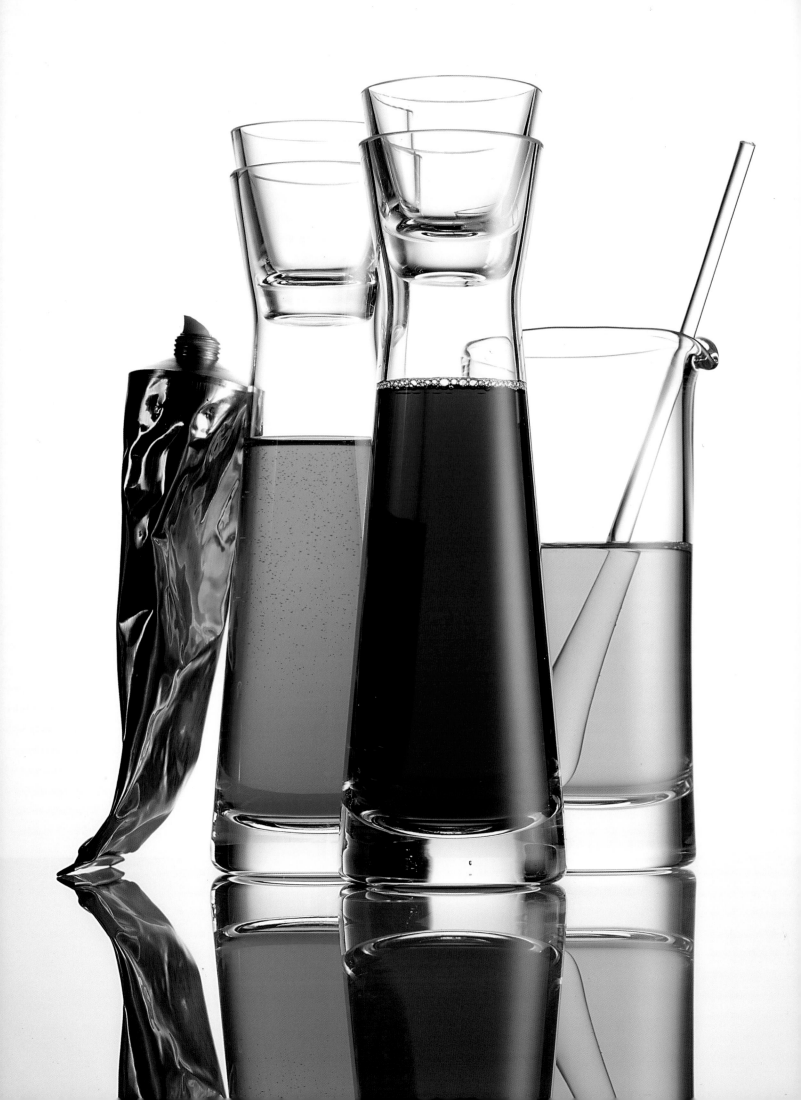

HAIR COLOR

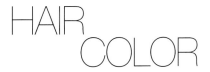

TEMPORARY COLORS Usually in the form of mousse, hairspray or shampoo, these coat the cuticles, forming a film of temporary color in an instant which will rinse out when the hair is washed. They are designed for minor changes to darken the tone of or intensify your natural color but unless specified do not have the ability to lighten the hair or conceal gray hair. Seek your stylist's advice before using on hair that is already color-treated or permed. Ash-blonde and silver shades are useful to brighten gray or white hair that has become yellow or dingy.

SEMI-PERMANENTS Like temporary colorants, semi-permanents coat the hair shaft with color pigments, but they last between five and seven washes, depending on how porous your hair is. If your hair is dry and damaged, it will absorb some of the color pigments, so the color will wash out less easily. Semi-permanent colors will not turn dark hair blonde but are ideal for enhancing your natural color, adding shine and concealing gray and experimenting without being stuck with the results for too long. This type of colorant should be applied to damp hair, which is shampooed once the color has developed.

DEMI-PERMANENTS These are longer-lasting versions of semi-permanent color which gradually fade between twelve and twenty washes. They penetrate the hair shaft slightly (so there can be signs of regrowth at the roots) and have more staying power, but they cannot lighten the hair. They are recommended for enhancing natural hair color, making hair a deeper color or covering hair that is up to 60 percent gray.

PERMANENT COLOR This type of colorant, which won't wash out, is available in several forms. First, there is henna, a natural long-lasting dye that can be removed only by cutting, which literally stains the hair. Then there are metallic dyes, which able to banish gray. They deposit metallic dyes and salts from various metals, such as silver, cobalt, copper and magnesium, on the hair shaft. Finally, there are chemical dyes or tints, which are the most commonly used form of permanent color and come in the widest range of colors. They work by opening up the cuticles so the color pigments enter the cortex. After the color has developed, the cuticles are closed, thus trapping in the color pigments permanently. This type of treatment will allow you to tint your hair up to four shades lighter than your natural color. The only drawback with permanent tints is that, as the hair grows, the roots will need retouching—usually every six to eight weeks.

BLEACHING If you want all your hair lightened or are looking for results that cannot be achieved with high-lift tint, you can bleach your hair. The strong alkaline solution used in bleaching raises the cuticles and the bleach will lighten the hair's natural pigments. Each hair goes through a color change from black to dark brown, red brown, golden brown, golden blonde and light blonde as the bleaching agents lighten the pigments. Rinsing stops the process at the shade you require. Leave this job to the experts, as color changes can be unpredictable. Due to the harsh chemical processing involved, hair can break easily and the product can burn the scalp if left on too long. If your scalp is prone to sensitivity, bleaching is not recommended. As it is the harshest of the color processes, you should follow a conditioning and restructuring after-care regimen. Semi-permanent colors can be applied to bleached hair to add color and help improve its condition.

HIGHLIGHTS AND LOWLIGHTS By using bleach or tint to highlight your hair, you can weave in up to three different tones of color to create an effect similar to sun-kissed lightening. Or, you can add contrasting shades to your natural color for a more striking effect. Lowlights can introduce deeper glints to the hair, darkening it in places or adding intensely toned colors such as copper, gold and red, which look great on dark blonde, brown and even black hair. As your hair grows, the roots will need retouching, probably after six or eight weeks.

COLOR CHOICE

Hair color, like makeup, must suit your complexion. Any hair color will look good with pale or ivory-colored skin. Women with pink skin should avoid shades of red or golden blonde, opting for ash tones to neutralize their coloring. Those with more sallow complexions should avoid yellow, gold or orange tones, going for deep reds and burgundies. Black skin will be complemented by colors similar to the natural hair color, although golden or red highlights can be striking. Those with olive skin tones should stay dark, adding richness to their hair with lowlights in red or brown shades, like chestnut or burgundy.

ON TRIAL

If you want to see the end results before you undergo a color change, cut off a tiny piece of hair close to the roots. Use a piece of sticky tape to hold the strands together at one end, then apply the color mixture. Leave on for the specified time, rinse out and wait until the hair is dry, then judge the results. This is a particularly good idea if your hair has already gone through chemical processing and is colored or permed, as the end results can be unpredictable. Or, to see what different hair colors will look like against your skin, try on wigs and hairpieces in shades you are considering.

DOS AND DON'TS

Never use tints, especially permanent ones, over henna, as there could be an adverse chemical reaction—leaving you with a hair color you never expected. Mix up the color before applying and then discard after using, unless the manufacturer's instructions suggest it will be safe to use again at a later date. Always use plastic rather than metal tools when mixing color. If you have had a perm, wait at least forty-eight hours before using a colorant. You should get your hair cut or reshaped after chemical processing, as even the healthiest hair will be porous around the ends and show damage.

TEST RUN

If you have never colored your hair before, always try a test patch for sensitivity before you start. Wipe a small section of skin behind your ear with an astringent-soaked cotton ball and then dab on a little hair tint using a cotton swab. Reapply two or three times, allowing the tint to dry between each application. Don't wash the area for forty-eight hours. After this time, if there is no skin redness or itching, the product will be safe to use. Never try shading the eyebrows or tinting the eyelashes with hair colorants. Because they are not formulated for use on sensitive areas, you could suffer an adverse reaction.

CLEAN UP

If you are not a professional applying color at home, follow these simple steps to make the task easier. Rub Vaseline into the skin around the hairline before applying color to act as a protective barrier and prevent staining of the skin. To remove after color processing, massage a small amount of cream cleanser into the Vaseline and then wipe off with a damp cotton ball. Always wear gloves while applying color and wrap a old dark-colored towel around your shoulders. If you get color in your eyes, rinse with lots of water immediately, and if irritation or reactions persist consult your doctor.

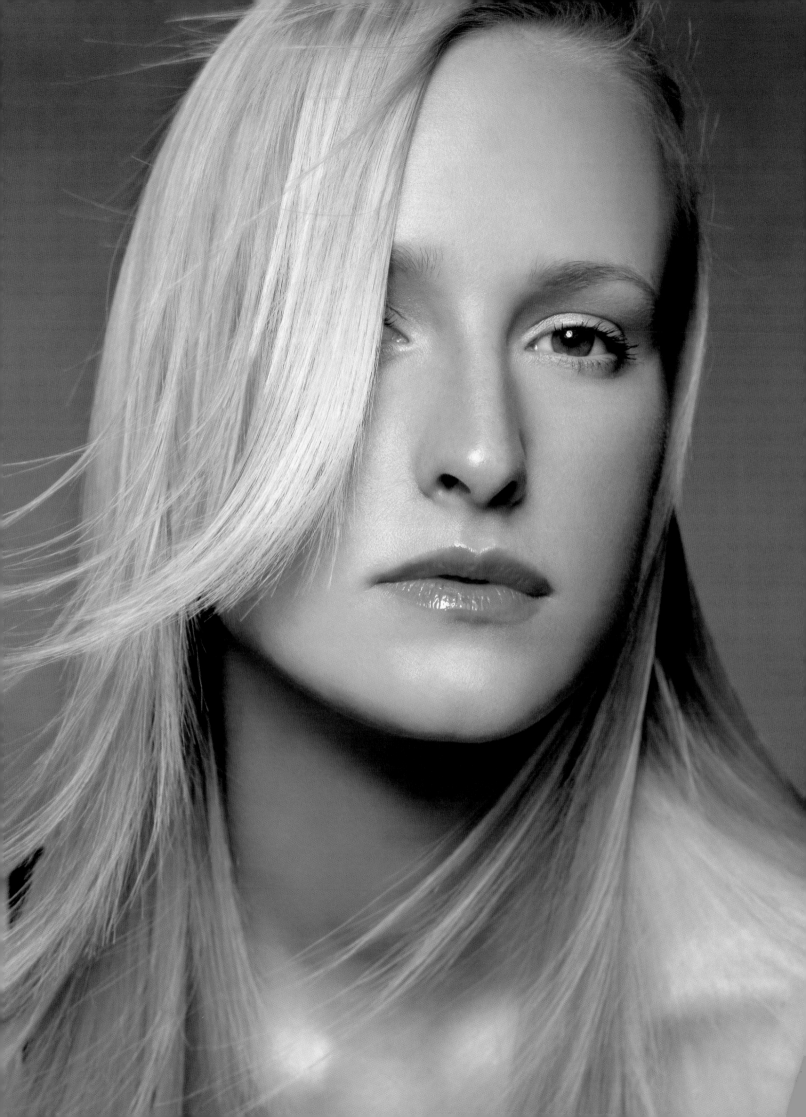

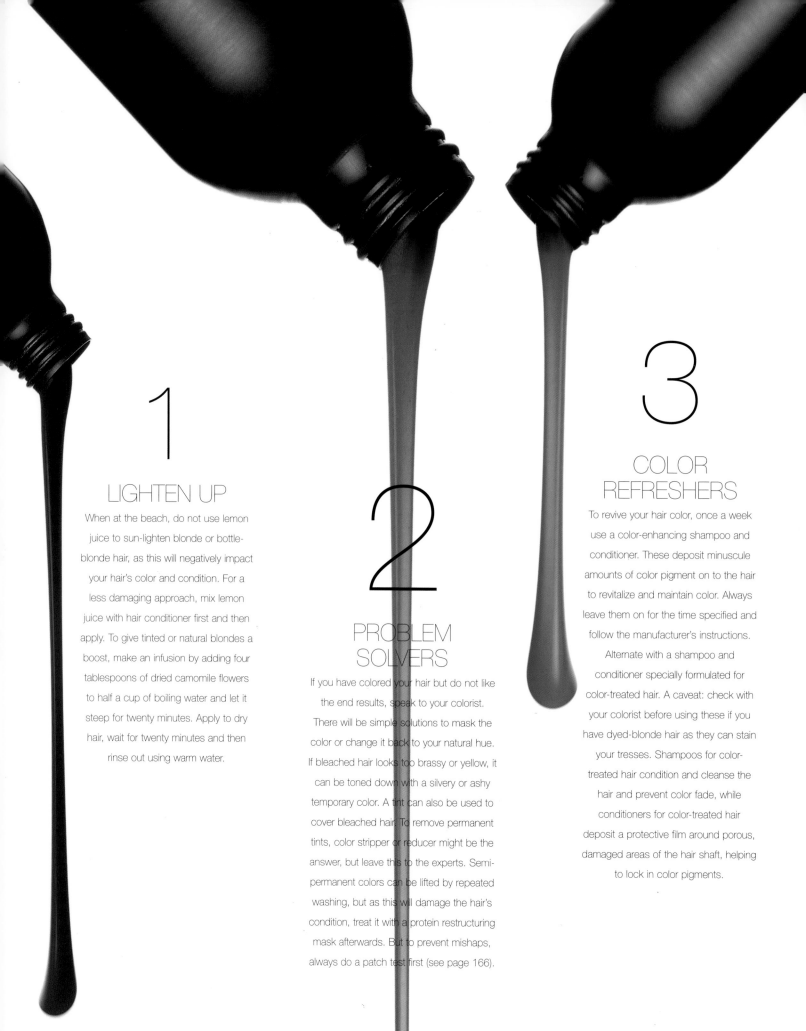

1

LIGHTEN UP

When at the beach, do not use lemon juice to sun-lighten blonde or bottle-blonde hair, as this will negatively impact your hair's color and condition. For a less damaging approach, mix lemon juice with hair conditioner first and then apply. To give tinted or natural blondes a boost, make an infusion by adding four tablespoons of dried camomile flowers to half a cup of boiling water and let it steep for twenty minutes. Apply to dry hair, wait for twenty minutes and then rinse out using warm water.

2

PROBLEM SOLVERS

If you have colored your hair but do not like the end results, speak to your colorist. There will be simple solutions to mask the color or change it back to your natural hue. If bleached hair looks too brassy or yellow, it can be toned down with a silvery or ashy temporary color. A tint can also be used to cover bleached hair. To remove permanent tints, color stripper or reducer might be the answer, but leave this to the experts. Semi-permanent colors can be lifted by repeated washing, but as this will damage the hair's condition, treat it with a protein restructuring mask afterwards. But to prevent mishaps, always do a patch test first (see page 166).

3

COLOR REFRESHERS

To revive your hair color, once a week use a color-enhancing shampoo and conditioner. These deposit minuscule amounts of color pigment on to the hair to revitalize and maintain color. Always leave them on for the time specified and follow the manufacturer's instructions. Alternate with a shampoo and conditioner specially formulated for color-treated hair. A caveat: check with your colorist before using these if you have dyed-blonde hair as they can stain your tresses. Shampoos for color-treated hair condition and cleanse the hair and prevent color fade, while conditioners for color-treated hair deposit a protective film around porous, damaged areas of the hair shaft, helping to lock in color pigments.

six secrets for color maintenance

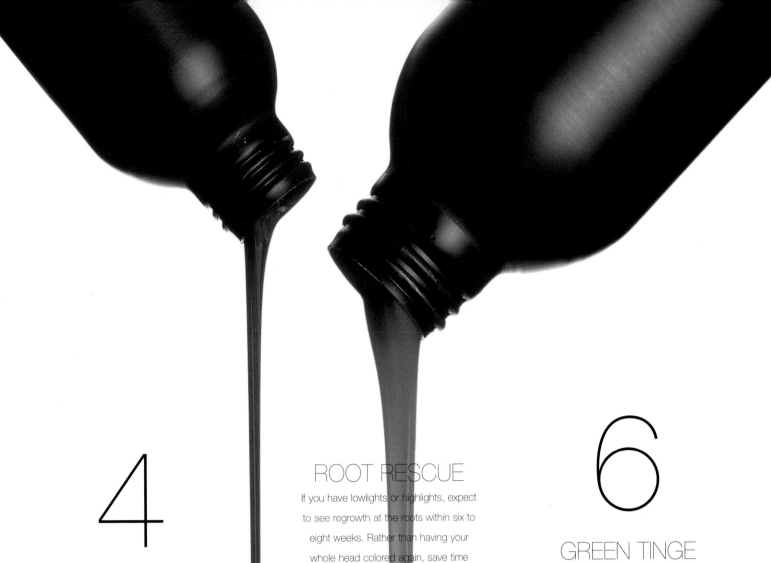

4

AFTER-CARE

Even though modern colorants are kind to the hair, chemical processing means that hair will require gentle handling. Don't overbrush it or use too many heated styling appliances. To help restore the strength and condition of your hair, use extra-nourishing and leave-in conditioners regularly. When you wash your hair, always finish off by rinsing with cold water, as this will close the cuticles, ensuring that they lie flat, which helps makes hair look shiny.

ROOT RESCUE

If you have lowlights or highlights, expect to see regrowth at the roots within six to eight weeks. Rather than having your whole head colored again, save time and money by asking your colorist to do just your hairline, crown and part. Also ask about different highlighting techniques that are easier to maintain. Traditional foil highlights and lowlights require precision application, which can make them costly and time-consuming, whereas widely spaced, less structured slices of color are much easier to retouch or change.

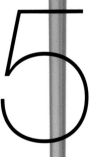

6

GREEN TINGE

If you have bleached or blonde-tinted hair, swimming in chlorinated water can turn it an unsightly shade of green. Basically, the chemicals in the water oxidize hair color. To prevent this, use products designed to protect the hair in chlorinated water and always rinse hair immediately after swimming. If your hair does have a green tinge, either book in to see your colorist or follow this correcting method: pour tomato juice on to the hair, massage it in, leave for a couple of minutes and then rinse out. The tomato juice will neutralize the green color and help restore both natural and dyed blondes to their former glory.

COLORADVICE

HENNA HELP
Think carefully before using henna to color your hair. It can give unpredictable results, can't be removed without cutting your hair and can't be used with other colorants, as the organic minerals it contains can react disastrously with them. The only way to improve a bad henna job is by using a chemical-free semi-permanent color, but consult your colorist first.

COLOR FADE
Try to color your hair four to six weeks before going on a sun-filled vacation so the sun's rays won't alter your new hue. Since sunlight works on the hair like peroxide, lifting the color and accelerating dryness and damage, protect your hair by applying preparations that are enriched with UV filters—or simply spread some sunscreen on your hair.

BRUNETTE BOOST
You don't need to spend big bucks on color-enhancing products. Try brewing a double espresso, letting it cool, and then using it as an infusion: pour over dry hair, wait thirty minutes and rinse. Or, steep two teaspoons of walnut leaves and a regular teabag in warm water. Let cool, then use as a post-shampooing rinse for dark hair.

COMING CLEAN
If you've colored your hair at home and stained your skin, rub the stained area with a cotton ball soaked with alcohol-based toner, or scrub with hot soapy water and a nailbrush. Some experts advise massaging whitening toothpaste into the skin, leaving it for five minutes and then removing with a tissue.

all you need to know about colorants

NATURAL COLOR

Certain hair colors will suit your natural color better than others. If your hair is dark to light brown, add streaks—go dark or red; if it's black, avoid going blonde or red; if it's dark to light blonde, opt for warm shades from honey to milky brown and chestnut; if it's gray/blonde, opt for pale, cool tones; and if it's gray, avoid going red.

COLOR PRECAUTIONS

Doubts exist about the safety of permanent and semi-permanent colorants for pregnant women, so avoid coloring methods that apply dye directly to the scalp and go instead for low- or highlights or a vegetable color. After three months, as hormonal changes improve your hair's condition, you may decide not to use color anyway.

COVER-UP

When melanin production stops, the hair becomes white, although this is perceived as gray. If you have up to 60 percent gray hair, try a demi-permanent color, which will last up to twenty washes. If you are above 60 percent gray, consider a permanent color. If you are happy with your natural gray, use a color-enhancing shampoo to bring out the silver tones.

VEGETABLE DYES

Made from natural extracts, vegetable dyes literally stain the hair when shampooed in and will last up to six washes. They boost natural shine and revitalize dull-looking locks but will not conceal gray. If you have bleached or color-treated hair, the results can be unpredictable; if hair is dry and damaged, the color will remain true for longer.

BEAUTY INTELLIGENCE

1 After coloring, do not expose your hair to chlorinated water or strong sunlight for forty-eight hours, as it will interfere with the results and your hair's condition.

2 If you have fine hair, remember that using permanent color can make it appear thicker, as the chemical processing involved will cause the hair shaft to swell.

3 If you have used a semi-permanent color on your hair but you don't like the results, use a clarifying or body-building shampoo to fade color quickly.

4 If you have greasy locks, the experts recommend using a hair colorant, because the chemical processes involved will change the natural porosity of your hair.

5 Keep in mind the color of your eyes and brows before opting for a color change. If you've lightened your hair, ask your colorist to lift your brow color too.

By adding highlights or lowlights you will break up the heaviness of very thick hair; they will also enhance fine hair by creating greater texture and more body.

6

7

Your hair color choice is vital: if the color is too light, it can make the hair look thinner, while rich tones will reflect more light and make it look much thicker.

To brighten your complexion, add a few subtle highlights to the hair around your face. Opt for tones that warm the skin and enhance your natural hair color.

8

If you have short hair, steer clear of highlights as they can result in a leopard-spotted effect. For the best results, try using a semi-permanent or permanent color.

9

You should treat colored hair to a hydrating mask once a week to replace lost moisture, but avoid hot-oil treatments, as they may strip out hair color.

10

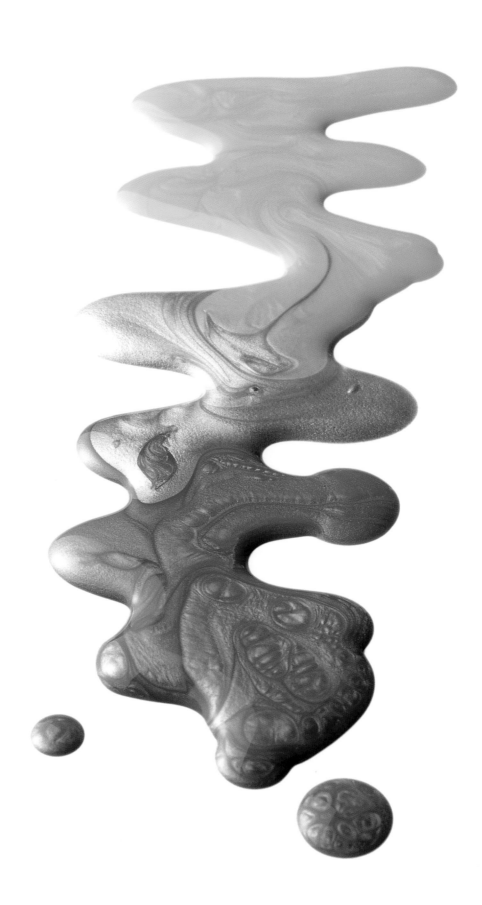

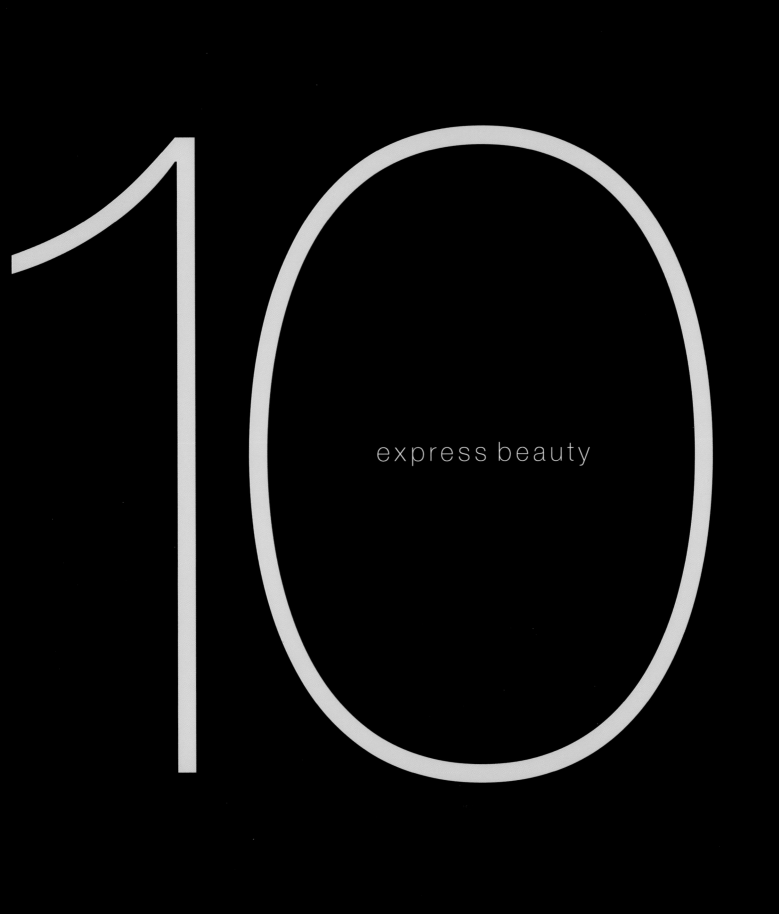

10

express beauty

You can get great results at high speed without sacrificing your looks. Try these quick-fix makeup tips, time-saving hair solutions and short cuts to good grooming. Then you'll have more time to enjoy life while still knowing you look your best.

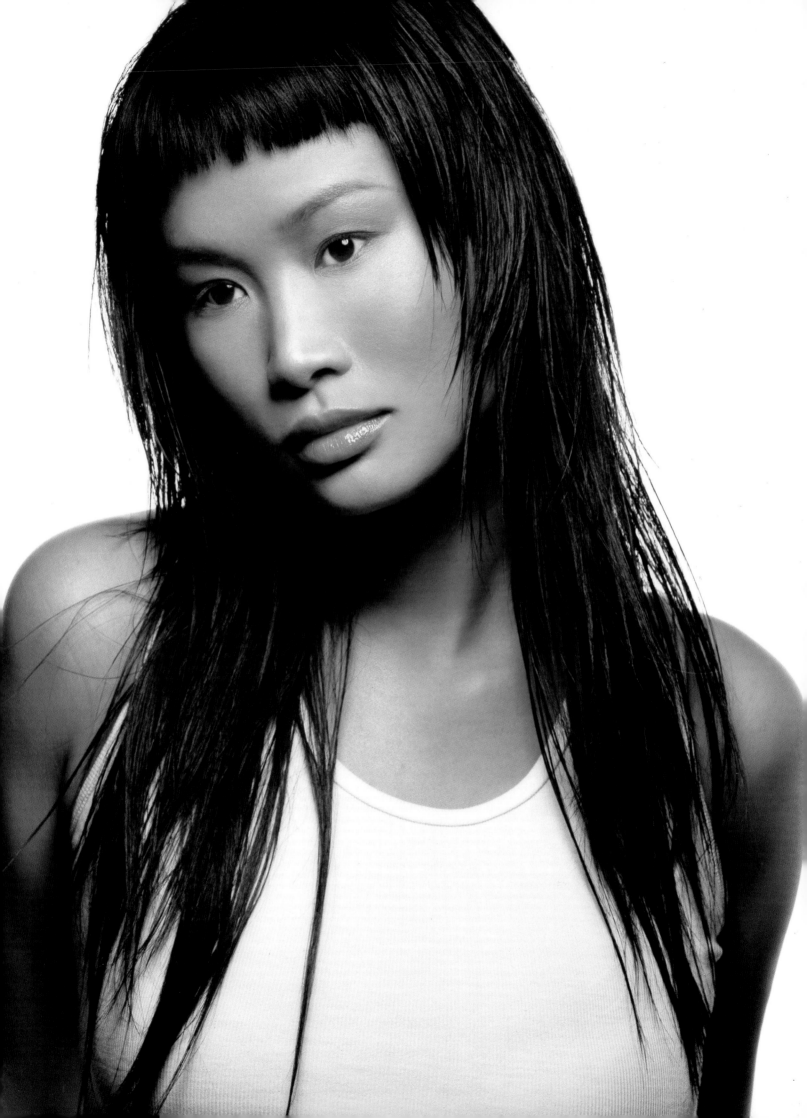

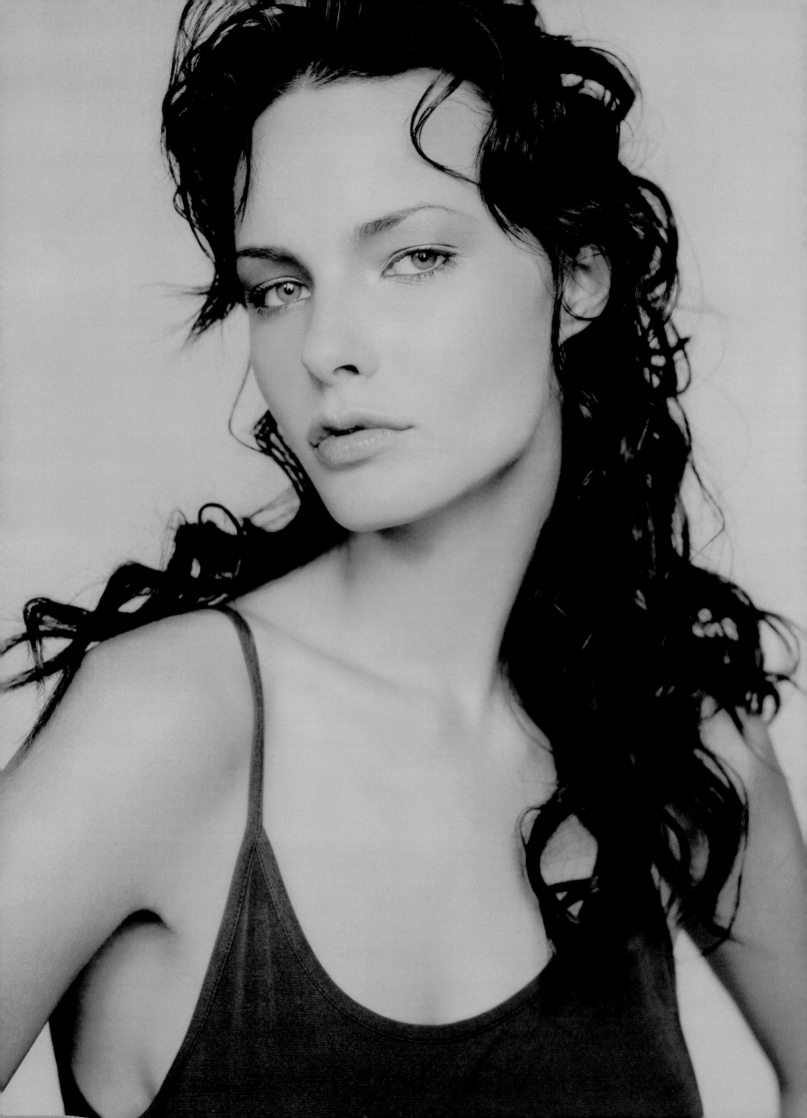

DOUBLE DUTY

Always choose dual-purpose beauty products to save time, or find ways to get more mileage from items you already have in your cosmetic collection when you're racing against the clock.

LIPSTICK Creamy lipsticks in soft shades of pink or rose can double as blush. Simply dot them on to the apples of your cheeks and then blend thoroughly into the skin, working in small circular motions, to produce a natural, healthy-looking finish.

EYESHADOW Let your eyeshadow work as eyeliner too by dampening a fine-tipped makeup brush with water, then dipping it in the eyeshadow and painting it along your lash lines.

MASCARA Clear mascara can be used to define the eyelashes and swept through the brows to tame unruly hairs.

PENCIL Invest in a neutral-colored pencil—for example, a taupe—and use it to add definition to the eyebrows, to outline the eyes and to shade the lips before coating with gloss.

BLUSH You can get more from a natural shade of cream blush by using it as a lip and eye color as well.

BRONZER Use bronzing powder not only to give the face a radiant finish but also to define the eyes, and to give a healthy glow to the rest of the body.

MOISTURIZER If you can't get to your stylist for a trim, try this quick fix: run an oil-based moisturizer through the ends of the hair to temporarily seal split ends.

CONCEALER As well as disguising any blemishes and imperfections, concealer can be used as a fixative for eyeshadow. Dab it over your eyelids with a fingertip, then apply your shadow as you normally would.

NAIL POLISH REMOVER In addition to lifting polish off nails, nail polish remover can help erase light stains (from spilled juice or smeared lipcolor) on your non-wood bathroom or kitchen counters and floors. Just dampen a paper towel with a little remover, then swipe.

SHAMPOO Mild shampoos are the perfect travelling companion. As well as handling your hair, they can be used to wash your body and even your clothes. When pressed for time, you can also choose an all-in-one shampoo and conditioner.

CONDITIONER Not only does conditioner detangle and soften your hair, it can also be used to smooth dry cuticles, cracked heels and rough elbows. Just massage it in as you would regular hand and body lotion.

SERUM During the summer, you can give bare legs a flattering, shiny finish by smoothing hair serum into the skin. Serums that have been enriched with ultraviolet protectors will also help guard the skin against damage from the sun's rays.

WAX If you are wearing leather shoes and suddenly notice that they are scuffed and in need of a shine but you don't have any polish on hand, you can massage hair wax or Vaseline into the leather to add shine, soften and buff.

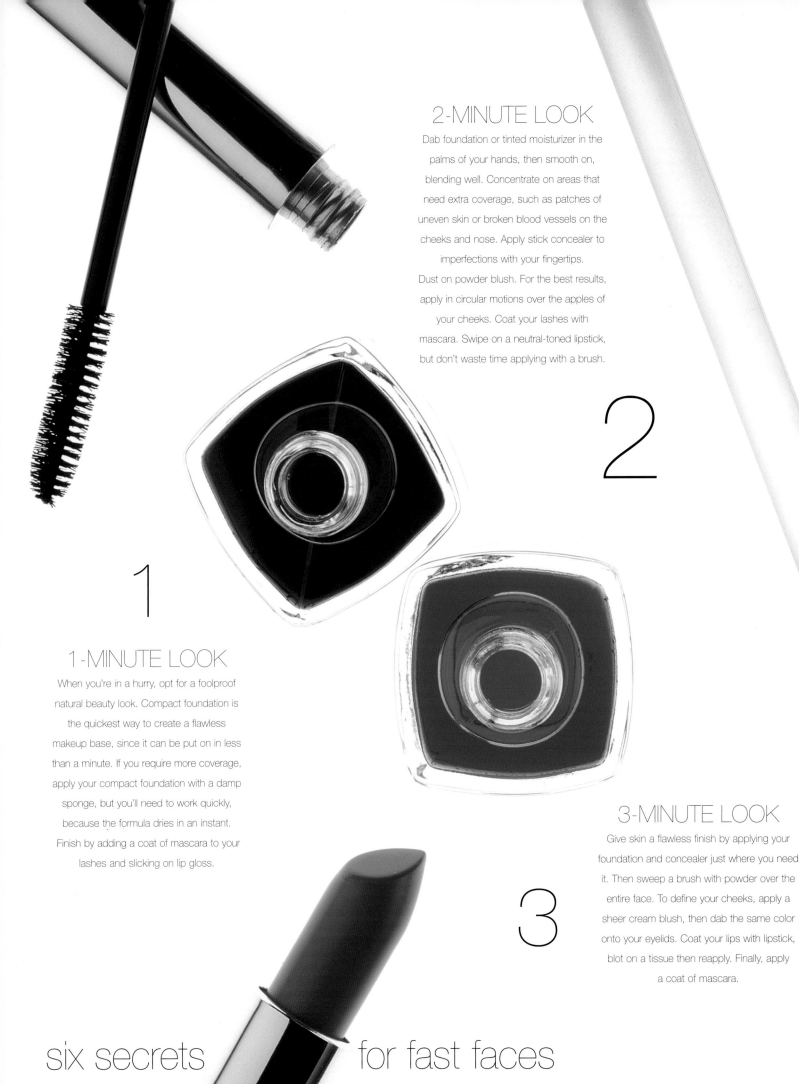

2-MINUTE LOOK

Dab foundation or tinted moisturizer in the palms of your hands, then smooth on, blending well. Concentrate on areas that need extra coverage, such as patches of uneven skin or broken blood vessels on the cheeks and nose. Apply stick concealer to imperfections with your fingertips. Dust on powder blush. For the best results, apply in circular motions over the apples of your cheeks. Coat your lashes with mascara. Swipe on a neutral-toned lipstick, but don't waste time applying with a brush.

2

1

1-MINUTE LOOK

When you're in a hurry, opt for a foolproof natural beauty look. Compact foundation is the quickest way to create a flawless makeup base, since it can be put on in less than a minute. If you require more coverage, apply your compact foundation with a damp sponge, but you'll need to work quickly, because the formula dries in an instant. Finish by adding a coat of mascara to your lashes and slicking on lip gloss.

3-MINUTE LOOK

Give skin a flawless finish by applying your foundation and concealer just where you need it. Then sweep a brush with powder over the entire face. To define your cheeks, apply a sheer cream blush, then dab the same color onto your eyelids. Coat your lips with lipstick, blot on a tissue then reapply. Finally, apply a coat of mascara.

3

six secrets   for fast faces

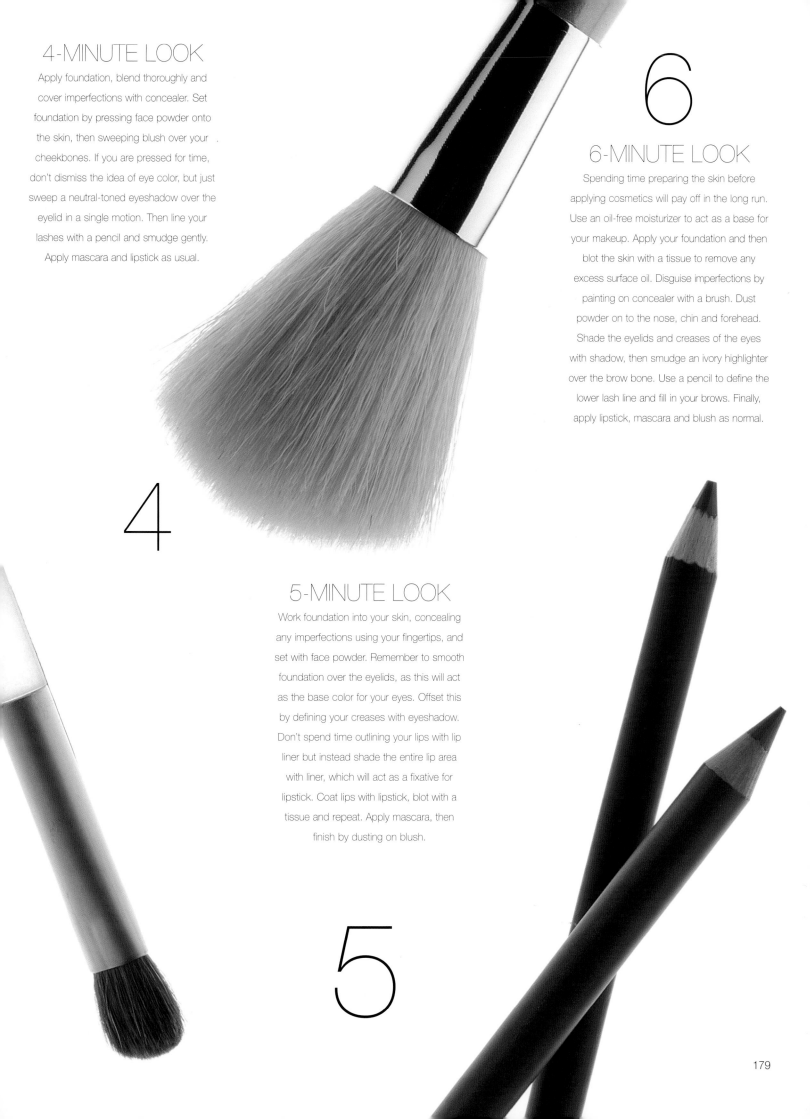

4-MINUTE LOOK

Apply foundation, blend thoroughly and cover imperfections with concealer. Set foundation by pressing face powder onto the skin, then sweeping blush over your cheekbones. If you are pressed for time, don't dismiss the idea of eye color, but just sweep a neutral-toned eyeshadow over the eyelid in a single motion. Then line your lashes with a pencil and smudge gently. Apply mascara and lipstick as usual.

6

6-MINUTE LOOK

Spending time preparing the skin before applying cosmetics will pay off in the long run. Use an oil-free moisturizer to act as a base for your makeup. Apply your foundation and then blot the skin with a tissue to remove any excess surface oil. Disguise imperfections by painting on concealer with a brush. Dust powder on to the nose, chin and forehead. Shade the eyelids and creases of the eyes with shadow, then smudge an ivory highlighter over the brow bone. Use a pencil to define the lower lash line and fill in your brows. Finally, apply lipstick, mascara and blush as normal.

4

5-MINUTE LOOK

Work foundation into your skin, concealing any imperfections using your fingertips, and set with face powder. Remember to smooth foundation over the eyelids, as this will act as the base color for your eyes. Offset this by defining your creases with eyeshadow. Don't spend time outlining your lips with lip liner but instead shade the entire lip area with liner, which will act as a fixative for lipstick. Coat lips with lipstick, blot with a tissue and repeat. Apply mascara, then finish by dusting on blush.

5

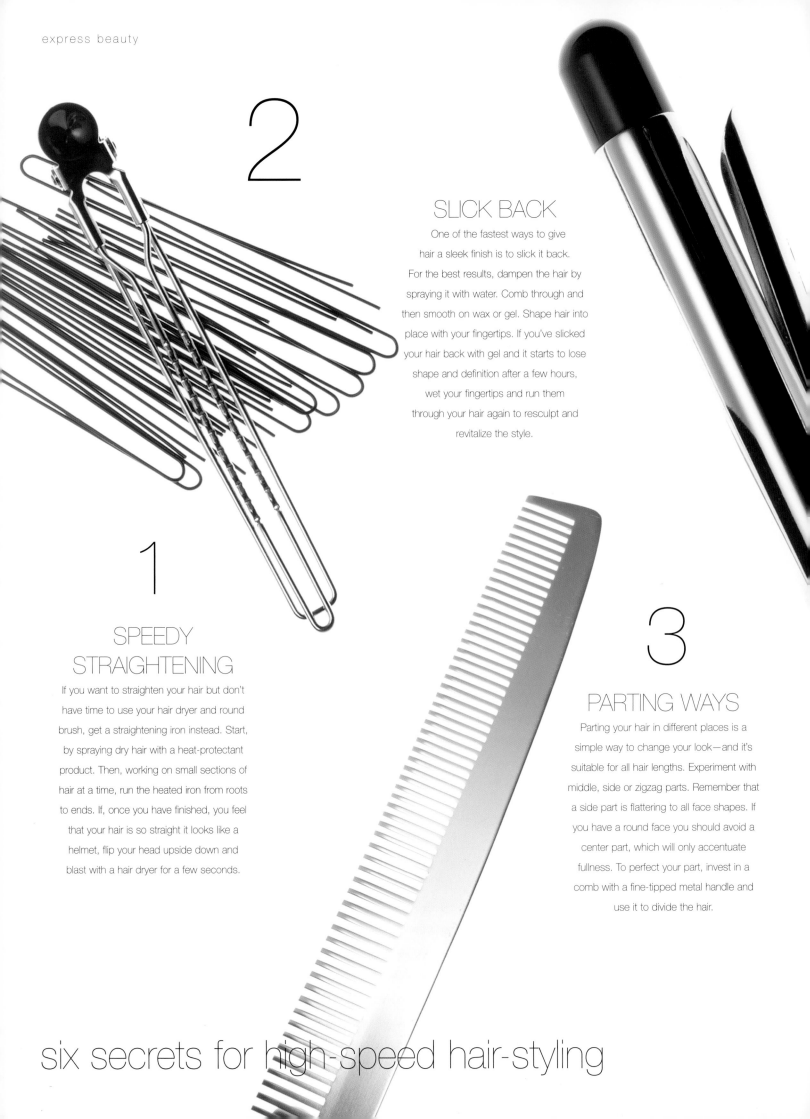

2

SLICK BACK

One of the fastest ways to give hair a sleek finish is to slick it back. For the best results, dampen the hair by spraying it with water. Comb through and then smooth on wax or gel. Shape hair into place with your fingertips. If you've slicked your hair back with gel and it starts to lose shape and definition after a few hours, wet your fingertips and run them through your hair again to resculpt and revitalize the style.

1

SPEEDY STRAIGHTENING

If you want to straighten your hair but don't have time to use your hair dryer and round brush, get a straightening iron instead. Start, by spraying dry hair with a heat-protectant product. Then, working on small sections of hair at a time, run the heated iron from roots to ends. If, once you have finished, you feel that your hair is so straight it looks like a helmet, flip your head upside down and blast with a hair dryer for a few seconds.

3

PARTING WAYS

Parting your hair in different places is a simple way to change your look—and it's suitable for all hair lengths. Experiment with middle, side or zigzag parts. Remember that a side part is flattering to all face shapes. If you have a round face you should avoid a center part, which will only accentuate fullness. To perfect your part, invest in a comb with a fine-tipped metal handle and use it to divide the hair.

six secrets for high-speed hair-styling

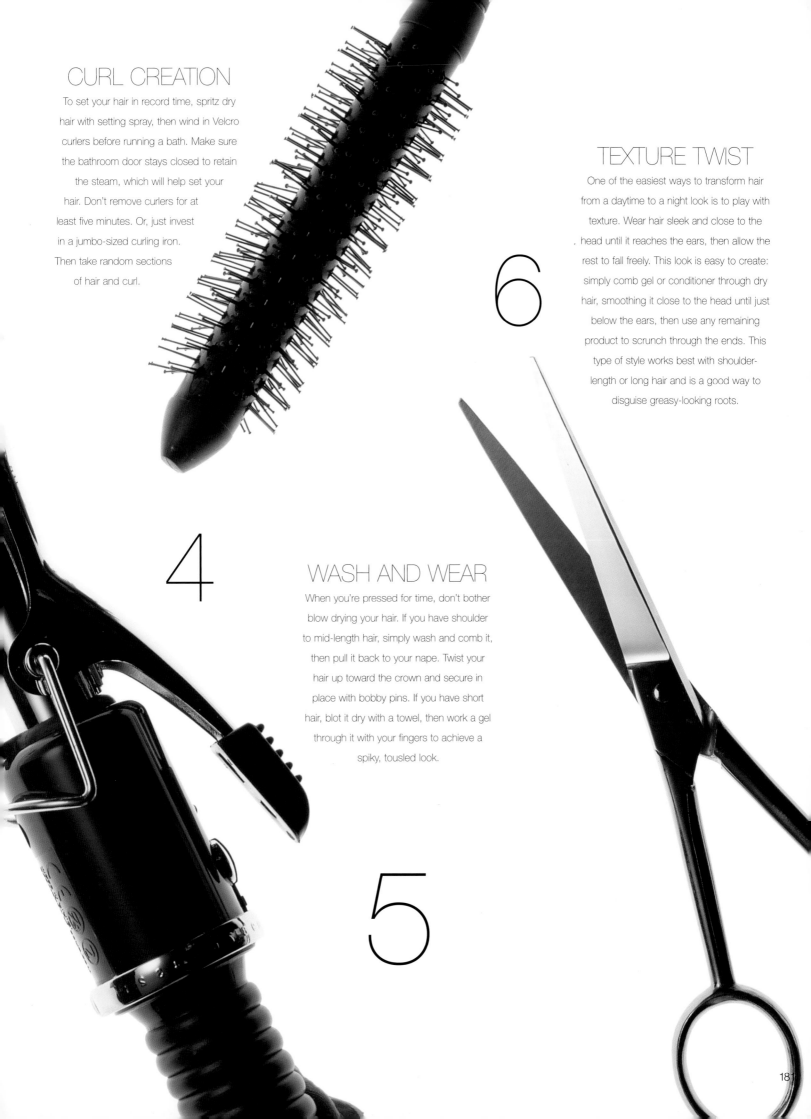

CURL CREATION

To set your hair in record time, spritz dry hair with setting spray, then wind in Velcro curlers before running a bath. Make sure the bathroom door stays closed to retain the steam, which will help set your hair. Don't remove curlers for at least five minutes. Or, just invest in a jumbo-sized curling iron. Then take random sections of hair and curl.

TEXTURE TWIST

One of the easiest ways to transform hair from a daytime to a night look is to play with texture. Wear hair sleek and close to the head until it reaches the ears, then allow the rest to fall freely. This look is easy to create: simply comb gel or conditioner through dry hair, smoothing it close to the head until just below the ears, then use any remaining product to scrunch through the ends. This type of style works best with shoulder-length or long hair and is a good way to disguise greasy-looking roots.

6

4

WASH AND WEAR

When you're pressed for time, don't bother blow drying your hair. If you have shoulder to mid-length hair, simply wash and comb it, then pull it back to your nape. Twist your hair up toward the crown and secure in place with bobby pins. If you have short hair, blot it dry with a towel, then work a gel through it with your fingers to achieve a spiky, tousled look.

5

INSTANTBEAUTY

PERFECT POUT

To smooth out chapped or dry lips before applying lipstick, coat them with petroleum jelly, then rub them gently with a toothbrush. Or, if you're short on time, just crack open a capsule of Vitamin E gel and use your finger to massage the serum into your lips.

CLEAVAGE ENHANCER

If you are going to wear a plunging neckline, makeup artists recommend that you use a bronze lipstick to enhance your cleavage. Draw a vertical line down the cleavage, then blend into the skin with the fingertips. This will create the illusion that your cleavage is bigger than it really is and will also give the skin a flattering finish.

HAIR VOLUMIZER

If your hair lacks body, sprinkle a little baby powder on your roots, flip your hair upside down and gently shake the hair with your fingers to distribute the powder down the hair shaft. Flip back up and lightly douse your head with soft-hold hairspray.

LUMINOUS SKIN

If your skin needs a pick-me-up, pep up your circulation by massaging in a moisturizer or foundation. For maximum impact, apply with gentle patting motions. This will help jump-start blood flow and make the skin look more radiant. Also, put your moisturizer in the fridge for several minutes before applying to give your skin an invigorating boost.

beautifying tips with immediate results

COLOR RETOUCH

If you have a few strands of gray hair that you want retouched, but don't have time to visit your colorist, you can temporarily disguise the problem yourself. Use mascara in the shade closest to your hair color to coat the strands of gray. This will be removed by washing your hair or brushing the color out.

MOISTURE BOOST

To help disguise wrinkles and fine lines, spray your face with a fine mist of water before smoothing on moisturizer. The cells in the skin's upper layers will absorb the water, making them look plumper, and this will make fine lines and wrinkles appear less prominent. Applying moisturizer afterwards will seal the water in, so the effect will last longer.

CUTICLE CARE

If you have unsightly pieces of stray skin around your cuticles, make them look more presentable in an instant by massaging the nail and cuticle with Vaseline. This will also give the nails a high-shine finish. If your fingertips feel greasy afterwards, either wipe with a tissue or use the excess product to tame split ends and give the hair shine.

EYE BENEFIT

Dermatologists are horrified at the thought, but many makeup artists in the film industry will arrive at a shoot armed with a tube of Preparation H. Normally used in the treatment of hemorrhoids, professionals swear it's a quick-fix solution for puffiness around the eyes. Smooth it on and wait: it is the best vasoconstrictor around, although it should only be used occasionally.

BEAUTY INTELLIGENCE

To prevent lip and eye pencils from crumbling and breaking when you sharpen them, place them in the fridge for ten minutes before use to harden.

Allowing your base coat and each layer of nail polish to harden for at least three minutes will help speed up drying time—and make chipping less likely.

If your eyes are puffy or irritated, try dabbing a cotton ball dampened with witch hazel beneath them—just be careful not to get the liquid in your eyes.

To quickly create a French-manicured effect, try running a white pencil under the nail tips, then painting the nails with a coat of clear or white nail polish.

Wearing peach or apricot blush will make all faces look youthful, whereas bluish-pink blush can have an aging affect.

Place a damp makeup sponge in the freezer for a few minutes, then roll it over your face to set makeup. It's also a great way to cool down when it's hot.

6

7

When applying mascara to your lower lashes, hold a tissue underneath to prevent mascara from collecting on your skin.

To make the whites of your eyes appear brighter, use a light blue pencil under the eyes. Soft blue eyeshadow lightly dusted just under the eyes will work too.

8

If you don't have a powder puff or brush with you for applying face powder, a cotton ball dipped in powder and pressed on to the skin will do the job.

9

10

Avoid metal nail files; they can tear soft or brittle nails. Instead, use only resin-coated emery boards, and file in just one direction (not back and forth).

GLOSSARY

ALKALINE
Substances with pH value between 7 and 14.

ALPHA HYDROXY ACIDS (AHAs)
A family of chemicals, including lactic acid and glycolic acid, that act by loosening (sloughing) dead skin cells from the skin's surface to uncover the fresher cells below.

ANTIOXIDANTS
Vitamins such as beta carotene, A and E, and substances such as green tea and grapeseed extract that counteract the damaging effects of free radicals, which accelerate the aging process.

CORTEX
Inner layer of the hair shaft that gives hair strength and elasticity. The source of the hair's color and curl.

CUTICLE
Outer layer of each strand of hair, made up of tiny, overlapping scales. If they don't lie flat, hair will look dull and be more prone to damage.

DERMIS
Second, thicker layer of skin below the epidermis.

EMOLLIENT
Ingredients in skin-care products that hydrate and soften the skin.

EPIDERMIS
Thin outer layer of the skin.

FOLLICLE
Hair follicles in the scalp's dermis are where all the nutrients and oxygen needed for healthy hair growth are found and all growth activity occurs.

FREE RADICALS
Rogue oxidants that are generated by sunlight, pollution, stress and smoking; they damage the skin by destabilizing its proper functioning.

HUMECTANT
Ingredients in cosmetic products that help the skin retain moisture.

HYALURONIC ACID
The skin's natural humectant that attracts water from the air and binds it to the skin. Cosmetic products contain it to help hydrate the skin.

HYPOALLERGENIC
Products that have been tested to ensure they won't cause allergic reactions, making them suitable for sensitive skin.

KERATIN
Protein found in hair, nails and skin.

MEDULLA
Core or central layer of hair shaft.

MELANIN
Skin and hair's natural pigment.

NON-COMEDEOGENIC
Products formulated to not clog pores, making them ideal for problem, blemish-prone skin.

PH
Scale that determines if a substance is acid or alkaline, ranging from 0 to 14. 7 is neutral, above 7 is alkaline and below 7 is acid.

PHEOMELANIN
Yellow/red pigments in the cortex that determine natural hair color.

PORES
Openings of sebaceous glands at skin's surface. Their size is inherited and blocked pores tend to be caused by sebum buildup.

POROUS
Hair that is dry, damaged and has undergone chemical processing is usually porous, meaning that it will quickly and unevenly absorb water or chemicals into the hair shaft.

RELAXED HAIR
Hair that has been chemically straightened.

SEBACEOUS GLANDS
Network of tiny glands that secrete sebum.

SEBUM
Oily, fatty substance formed in tiny glands around every hair on the body. It acts as a lubricant for skin and hair, and helps protect skin.

T-ZONE
Oily area of skin across the forehead, down the nose and on the chin.

INDEX

DEBBIE PIKE With a degree in graphics and a passion for fashion and beauty, Debbie Pike worked for ten years in London as an art director on magazines such as British *Elle*, *GQ* and *Esquire*. She then moved to Sydney and spent the next two years working on the launch of Australian *marie claire* and for a fashion advertising agency. In 1997 she relocated to New York, where she is now working as a freelance creative director, with many editorial and advertising clients.

DAVID PARFITT The photographs of London-based photographer David Parfitt have appeared in many editorial and advertising projects all over the world during the last fifteen years. Specializing in still-life photography, he is renowned for his innovative approach and ability to make inanimate objects appear exciting and desirable.

TROY WORD Troy Word's desire to be involved in the world of fashion photography took him from Bartlesville, Oklahoma, to the School of Visual Arts in New York City. After graduation and an internship with Albert Watson, he moved to Europe in order to develop his individual style and hone his photographic skills. Today, his work is highly respected worldwide, as indicated by his most recent cosmetic campaigns for Lancôme, Almay and Plenitude by L'Oréal.

Special thanks to Sam Girdwood, Kate Wililams, Sophie Peter, Abigail and Melissa at Shu Uemura, Carrie Kilpatrick, Suzie Cunningham, Emma, Nichole and Claire at Clinique, Sarah Griffith, Natalie Agussol, Daniel at Artomatic, Millie Kendall, Cassandra, Caroline and Susan at Lancôme, Natalie Buckley, Fiona, Owen and Tasia at Dowal Walker PR, Vic Hyde and Rosanna at L'Oréal, Sarah North, Trudi Collister, Grace and Lynette at Whistles, Kathryn Deighton at Muji, Mark Smith at Screen Face and the team at Astrid Sutton Associates, Riverhouse, Karen Berman PR and Felicity Calhrope PR.

Thank you for products and clothing for photography to Clinique, Shu Uemura, Chanel, Christian Dior, Yves Saint Laurent, Estée Lauder, Lancôme, Nars, Stila, Trish McEvoy, Laura Mercier, Issey Miyake, Spectacular, Prescriptives, Gucci, Club Monaco, Paul Mitchell, Bourjois, Iman, The Body Shop, Ruby Hammer, Diamancel, Tweezerman, Boots, No7, Hard Candy, L'Oréal, CP Hart, John Lewis, Original Source, Poppy, Origins, Penhaligons, Czech & Speake, Floris, Toni & Guy, Redken, Aveda, Helena Rubenstein, John Frieda, Charles Worthington, Bulgari, Oribe, L'Occitane, Revlon, BaByliss, Trucco, Vidal Sassoon, Elizabeth Arden, Guerlain, BeneFit, Face Stockholm, MAC, Rimmel, Neal's Yard, Pears, Annick Goutal, La Prairie, L'Clerc, Perfumes Isabell, Jil Sander, Shiseido, Clarins, Philosophy, Jo Malone, Virgin Vie, Crabtree & Evelyn, Bloom, Calvin Klein, Artomatic for their vacuum-packing services, John Smedley, Whistles, Saba, Muji, Aria and Screen Face.

Still-life photos by David Parfitt: back cover, pages 6, 8, 12, 14, 18, 22, 25, 26, 32, 36, 40, 42, 48, 68, 74, 78, 86, 90, 92, 96, 100, 103, 108, 112, 119, 128, 132, 136, 139, 144, 158, 162, 166, 172, 178, 180.

Beauty photos by Troy Word: front cover, pages 11, 17, 21, 35, 39, 51, 52, 55, 56, 59, 60, 61, 62, 63, 71, 72, 77, 81, 89, 95, 99, 111, 115, 116, 120, 123, 131, 135, 147, 148, 150, 151, 152, 153, 161, 165, 175, 176.